Epidemiologic Studies in Psychosomatic Medicine

Advances in Psychosomatic Medicine

Vol. 9

S. Karger · Basel · München · Paris · London · New York · Sydney

Epidemiologic Studies in Psychosomatic Medicine

Volume Editors
STANISLAV KASL, New Haven, Conn. and FRANZ REICHSMAN, Brooklyn, N.Y.

8 figures and 6 tables, 1977

S. Karger · Basel · München · Paris · London · New York · Sydney

Advances in Psychosomatic Medicine

Vol. 5: Training in Psychosomatic Medicine. XII + 180 p., 1967.
ISBN 3-8055-0459-4
Vol. 6: Duodenal Ulcer. X + 200 p., 14 fig., 11 tab., 1971.
ISBN 3-8055-1159-0
Vol. 7: Hunger and Satiety in Health and Disease. XII + 336 p., 31 fig., 14 tab., 1972.
ISBN 3-8055-1356-9
Vol. 8: Psychosocial Aspects of Physical Illness. XIV + 276 p., 17 fig., 4 tab., 1972.
ISBN 3-8055-1339-9

Cataloging in Publication
Epidemiologic studies in psychosomatic medicine / volume editor, Franz Reichsmann.
– Basel, New York: Karger, 1977.
(Advances in psychosomatic medicine; v. 9)
1. Psychophysiologic Disorders – occurrence I. Reichsman, Franz, ed. II. Title
III. Series
W1 AD81 v. 9 / WM 90 E64
ISBN 3-8055-2654-7

Printed in Switzerland by Buch- und Offsetdruckerei Kohlhepp AG, Allschwil
ISBN 3-8055-2654-7

Contents

Introduction

This is a slimmer volume than the editors had intended it to be: it proved impossible to get commitments for contributions from expert authors in certain areas of epidemiologic, psychosocial research in which sufficient or even abundant data had accumulated. Clearly, this is an expression of heavy commitments which investigators have made for years in advance; it includes workers who have studied specific diseases as well as those who have researched the relationships between stressful life situations on the one hand and morbidity and mortality on the other hand. In regard to one syndrome, anorexia nervosa, the volume is rich because it contains two chapters on this important illness. The editors do not consider this fact an embarrassment of riches because the chapters by Drs. CRISP and HILL do not lead to redundancy of material but complement each other.

Important objectives of this volume are: the distributing of knowledge concerning epidemiologic data and concepts as well as pointing to the many areas in which data obtained so far are sketchy or given to varying interpretations or almost nonexistent. Dr. KASL particularly, in his 'Summarizing Discussion', points lucidly to numerous questions which need much further exploration.

Last not least, we trust that the volume will provide leads for psychosomatic investigators to observe psychologically small groups of patients *in depth,* using as their take-off point data obtained by epidemiologic studies. In turn, the results of the in-depth studies should raise new questions and give leads to innovative epidemiologic research. We consider this sort of cross-fertilization an important source for productive investigations in psychosomatic medicine.

FRANZ REICHSMAN, MD
Professor of Medicine (assigned from Psychiatry)
Downstate Medical Center *Brooklyn, N.Y. 11203* (USA)

Adv. psychosom. Med., vol. 9, pp. 1–19 (Karger, Basel 1977)

Epidemiological Studies of the Psychosomatic Aspects of Coronary Heart Disease

A Review[1,2]

C. DAVID JENKINS

Department of Behavioral Epidemiology, Boston University School of Medicine, Boston, Mass.

Contents

Traditional epidemiological studies of coronary heart disease (CHD) have usually omitted consideration of dynamic variables of interest to psychosomatic workers, primarily due to the difficulty of measuring these variables reliably. On the other hand, psychosomatic studies have tended to be too small to be considered truly epidemiological because of the depth of

1 The background research and preparation of this paper was supported by Research Grant HL 15399 from the National Heart and Lung Institute of the US Dept. of Health, Education and Welfare. The author acknowledges with appreciation the editorial suggestions of Dr. STEPHAN J. ZYZANSKI and the technical assistance of Ms. SUSAN A. ZOELLER, Dept. of Behavioral Epidemiology, Boston University School of Medicine, and Ms. MARCIA FORD, MEDLARS Search Analyst, Countway Library, Harvard University School of Medicine.
2 Submitted for publication: September 1974

investigation required for a comprehensive examination of the variety of psychosomatic mechanisms that might be operating in patients and controls. Despite these obstacles to the combination of the best features of psychosomatic depth and epidemiological breadth, an impressive array of studies has been published recently, making CHD better investigated psychosomatically than perhaps any other chronic or infectious diesease, excluding psychiatric disorders.

Still, questions are often raised about the value of such efforts. For example, is it worthwhile to pursue the psychsomatic aspects of CHD? Have not epidemiologic studies of accepted risk factors like elevated blood pressure, high serum cholesterol, cigarette smoking, and overweight, adequately explained the etiology of this disease?

Recent epidemiologic studies using traditional risk factors reinforce the validity of the above variables, but also reveal that in combination they can explain only about half the variablility in CHD rates among population groups. A recent study by GARCIA-PALMIERI *et al.* [1972] comparing prevalence of coronary disease in Honolulu, Puerto Rico, and Framingham found that when the Framingham risk factor equation was applied to Honolulu or Puerto Rico, twice as many CHD cases were predicted to occur as were observed. Somehow the presence of the major risk factors, found so important in the continental United States, does not carry the same pathological consequences in either of these other social and geographic environments. A similar finding is reported by KEYS in applying multiple logistic risk factor equations from the US to European data and vice versa. US citizens have about twice the rate of CHD as Europeans with similar levels of these specific risk factors [KEYS *et al.,* 1972]. It should also be kept in mind that any one standard risk factor is not associated with CHD incidence or prevalence in all populations [see for example, KEYS, 1970]. Thus it would appear that although much is known about the precursors of CHD, at least an equal amount remains unknown. It is into this obscure area of CHD etiology that we must throw the searchlight of psychosomatic and epidemiologic study.

Comprehensive reviews of the literature studying the relationship of various psychosocial factors to coronary disease have appeared in recent years. MAI [1968] categorized the 55 papers he reviewed using an original organizing scheme. He concluded that both personality and stress may be involved in the pathogenesis of CHD, and that they might be more relevant to the development of angina pectoris than to myocardial infarction. CHRISTIAN [1968] organized his German-language review of European and United

States research into six categories of behavioral influences on CHD risk. A comprehensive French-language review was prepared by MERTENS and SEGERS [1971, part 1]. It summarizes the available literature through mid-1970, but on the whole is less optimistic about progress in the field than the English-language review of 162 papers prepared at about the same time by JENKINS [1971].

The present paper will attempt to cover the empiric research into psychological, social, and behavioral factors associated with risk of coronary heart disease which has appeared in serial publications since the time span covered by the reviews of MAI, CHRISTIAN, MERTENS and SEGERS, and JENKINS. The author depended heavily on the MEDLARS (medical literature analysis and retrieval service) of the USPHS National Library of Medicine. The coverage of journal articles in languages other than English is less adequate because some of these papers were not available to the author for review. The research studies will be grouped according to the following topical categories: (1) sociologic indexes; (2) social mobility and status incongruity; (3) anxiety and neuroticism; (4) life dissatisfactions; (5) stress and life change; (6) coronary-prone behavior pattern, and (7) other traits and defenses, such as denial and response sets.

Sociologic Indexes

The most striking differences in CHD incidence and mortality are found between populations of different countries. Here sociologic and geographic influences are combined. The monumental studies by KEYS and his colleagues from seven countries reveal wide ranges of rates of CHD incidence, prevalence, and mortality in different parts of the world [KEYS, 1970]. These differences are striking even though great care was taken to study well-defined population subgroups comprehensively and to perform all risk factor and diagnostic determinations using uniform methodology. For the seven countries studied the highest CHD rates in all age groups were found in Finland and the United States while the lowest rates were consistently found in Greece, Yugoslavia and Japan. Even lower rates appear to prevail in Nigeria, where a series of 8,000 necropsies revealed only 6 myocardial infarctions involving atherosclerosis [WILLIAMS, 1971].

One section of the KEYS report sought to separate the effects of socioeconomic status and amount of physical activity on risk of CHD. It was generally found that when amount of physical activity is statistically controlled, the remaining occupational differences in CHD rates are substantially larger than is the case for differences in CHD rates associated with physical activity when occupation is statistically controlled. This calls into question the validity of the conclusion by McDONOUGH *et al.* [1965] in Evans County, Georgia, where they attributed their observed differences in CHD prevalence between occupational groups to physical activity differences (without a direct attempt to disentangle these correlated variables). The Keys' work on seven large samples would suggest that occupation and its associated way of life contributes differentially to CHD risk above and beyond the physical labor involved in the job itself. It is important for future behavioral epidemiologic studies to discover the mechanisms of this relationship.

WEISS [1973] reviewed CHD mortality rates in the USA by marital status and also the distributions of traditional CHD risk factors in these statuses as determined by US Health Examination Survey. Despite substantial differences in CHD mortality among marital status categories, there were no consistent differences in cholesterol, blood pressure, or ponderal index between marital categories when large representative samples were examined. WEISS concludes: 'The attributes of nonmarried persons responsible for their excess CHD mortality remain obscure.' THIEL *et al.* [1973] in a retrospective matched sample study found a higher prevalence of divorce among men with myocardial infarction (MI). It appeared that sociologic or psychologic elements in their way of life may be contributing to these MI differences independent of traditional risk factors.

The relation of socioeconomic status (SES) and occupation to CHD incidence and mortality has been widely studied. The results point in conflicting directions. It may well be that the social stratum most at risk of CHD will be different at varying periods of a nation's evolution from rural-agrarian to industrialized society. The most recent survey by CASSEL *et al.* [1971] in a rural county in the southern US found a changed picture of CHD risk by SES level in 1969 as compared to their prevalence findings from 7 years earlier. Race and sex differences (white males as the singularly highest group) continued as before, but lower social class white males seem to be incurring increased CHD such that they are no longer significantly less affected than the middle and upper classes. SIGURJONSSON [1971] studying CHD mortality by occupation in Iceland found a higher proportion of all deaths attributable to CHD among white-collar workers as contrasted with farmers. This is partially influenced by competing causes of death, such as accidents and cancer, which are higher in farming, laboring and maritime occupations. A noteworthy difference in the basic CHD mortality remained, however, and the precise reasons for it are not known.

Another component of most indexes of social status is education. This has been shown to be related in complex ways to CHD risk, often because it is confounded with other aspects of social class [JENKINS, 1971]. A retrospective study of 250 male patients with MI by CROOG and LEVINE [1969] shows that education may operate through a psychosomatic avenue to influence self-report of clinical CHD symptoms. These workers found that among men with confirmed diagnoses of myocardial infarction, those with higher education were more likely to report the presence of chest pains before the actual acute episode than were men with lower education. Conversely, the latter group usually denied having any premonitory symptoms, and the few who did, often reported complaints in the gastrointestinal system. Future research is needed to determine whether these differences in symptom reporting are a function of differential thresholds of pain sensitivity, differential awareness of organ systems, or the operation of denial. It should be further determined why these are linked to level of education.

A quite different social interaction variable has been found related to CHD mortality by COMSTOCK and PARTRIDGE [1972] who performed a very thorough retrospective case-control study in Maryland. The intent of this team was to search for differences in CHD mortality associated with varying levels of water hardness. No such association was found, but a strong relationship between frequency of church attendance and risk of coronary death was observed. In men, frequent attenders of religious services had only 60% the mortality rate of those who rarely of never attended. For women, the corresponding figure was 50%. Thus in effect COMSTOCK has replicated the study on two independent population groups (the two sexes) in the same county. The hypothesis was entertained that perhaps the beginnings of illness reduced frequency of church attendance such that the decedents rarely attended. Various additional probes and approaches to data analysis tend to weaken this explanation. In addition, the authors report that a similar association between myocardial infarction and synagogue attendance was found by SHAMGAR and MEDALIE in Israel.

Social Mobility and Status Incongruity

Research covered in earlier reviews showed consensus that CHD risk was related to social mobility, both those changes occurring between generations and those within the lifetime of the group at risk. There was also evidence from several studies that CHD risk was related to status incongruity, the condition of possessing simultaneously the 'identifying markings' of different social classes, as evidenced by discrepancies between levels of education, occupation, income, quality of housing, organizational membership, etc. Status incongruity is evidence that certain aspects (but not all) of a person's life have experienced cultural mobility during his own lifetime. Studies published in the last 4 years have not included status incongruity as an independent variable and hence no further evaluation of it as a risk factor can be made. Several studies have included indexes of social mobility and their association with CHD has yielded conflicting evidence.

MEDALIE *et al.* [1973a] followed 10,000 Israeli government employees for 5 years documenting the occurrence of MI. They found sharp differences in rates of MI in immigrants by their country of birth. Lowest rates were in persons born in Middle Eastern countries outside of Israel. The highest were in immigrants from Europe. Intergenerational differences were also significant with intermediate rates occurring in immigrants, highest rates in those who were first generation Israeli (their fathers were born elsewhere), and lowest rates were found in second generation Israelis (both they and their fathers were born in Israel). This finding is not in keeping with the simpler hypothesis that a person's own life changes adversely affect his CHD risk.

WARDWELL and BAHNSON's [1973] Southeast Connecticut study also showed retrospectively that patients with MI had experienced less cultural mobility than the normal comparison group. Cultural mobility in this study was broadly defined as the summation of a variety of major changes in life situation, patterned generally after the definitions of SYME *et al.* [1965]. Analysis of occupational changes in the Western Collaborative Group Study showed that higher rates of CHD occurred prospectively more often in men with 0 or 1 job change in the past 10 years as contrasted to those with two or more job changes [WILLIAMS, 1968]. Most of these were minor changes and not shifts to a totally different occupational category, which was the criterion used by SYME. The Evans County studies of heart disease incidence and prevalence found during their 1969 resurvey that upward mobility had different implications for CHD prevalence depending upon the social class from which the respondent began his change and depending upon whether intergenerational or intragenerational mobility was being considered [KAPLAN *et al.*, 1971]. The numbers of cases were small in many key subgroups and no statistical tests were calculated, thus leaving these findings suggestive rather than conclusive.

One finding in positive support of the mobility hypothesis was reported by MEDALIE *et al.* [1973b] in their prospective study of Israeli men. Geographic mobility was found associated with the incidence of new angina pectoris in the 1,112 men who had lived in three or more countries since the age at which they started employment. This was the only aspect of mobility found in this study to be associated with CHD incidence.

The retrospective analysis by LEHR *et al.* [1973] conducted as part of the Western Collaborative Group Study, showed CHD prevalence in the study subjects to correlate at a low but significant level with (1) the discrepancy between the social status levels of their mother's versus their father's religious affiliation, (2) father's occupation, and (3) subject's income. This 'parental religious difference factor' suggests there may be some contribution to CHD risk which is associated with exposure to conflicting expectations in early childhood. This is generally consistent with the incongruity hypothesis.

Anxiety and Neuroticism

Much additional evidence has accumulated that anxiety, depression, other distressing feelings, and a variety of neurotic defenses against them are associated with angina pectoris and MI in retrospective and prospective studies. THIEL *et al.* [1973] studying 50 patients with MI and 50 age-matched controls found the MIs to score far higher on anxiety and depression scales, to report significantly more feelings of nervousness, sleep disturbances, and dyspnea. The significance of these differences may have been heightened by the comparison of MIs with healthy controls as contrasted with control groups of patients hospitalized with other diseases, as have been used in other studies, or may have been influenced by retrospective bias among the MI patients. Nevertheless, further probing of the patients' repsonses by THIEL and his co-workers revealed that many subjects reported having been anxious and depressed for considerable time prior to their MI. The report of sleep disturbances is confirmed by findings of the Kaiser-Permanente study [FRIEDMAN *et al.*, 1974] which found prospectively that persons who reported trouble falling asleep or staying asleep were more likely to be in a group who later developed MI than in a control group remaining free of CHD. Similarly, THOMAS and GREENSTREET [1973] studying medical school students found that those who reported being tired upon awakening later incurred MI more often. The Kaiser-Permanente study was based on Health Plan records wherein many thousands of subjects responded to a 155-item true-false questionnaire similar to parts of the Minnesota Multiphasic Personality Inventory (MMPI). Persons who later developed MI more often endorsed the series of items implying 'emotional drain' and 'somaticizing' (the conversion of unpleasant emotions into physical symptoms) than did persons remaining free of disease. The strength of these differences was reduced substantially when all persons with symptoms suggestive of possible myocardial ischemia at intake and their respective controls were removed from the sample. Nevertheless, this general finding receives further support from a study by KAVANAGH and SHEPARD [1973] who noted increased tiredness and poorer general health in the week before MI in 102 survivors of this event (no control group).

MERTENS and SEGERS [1971, part 2] report an association between anxiety and CHD, emphasizing the weakness of defense mechnasims. Their retrospective study, however was based on contrasts between urban patients with subjective symptoms and rural patients with medically determined signs of CHD. The approach to diagnosis is thus confounded with area of residence.

GREENE *et al.* [1972] report that sudden death is frequently preceded by a period of depression followed by an abrupt change to arousal marked by increased work, anxiety, or anger. This study can be seen as hypothesis-generating rather than hypothesis-testing in that it had no specific measures of these affects and no control group.

In a carefully matched case control study WARDWELL and BAHNSON [1973] found patients with MI to score much higher than other hospitalized patients and somewhat higher than normals on the scales for alienation and for total psychopathology, the latter included items for anxiety and a variety of disturbing emotions. MAYOU [1973] found angina patients to manifest more anxiety, depression, irritability, and sleeplessness than his contrast group. RUSKIN *et al.* [1970] studying 128 men in a Work Evaluation Unit showed these men to score higher than average on several MMPI scales particularly depression, hypochondriasis, and hysteria, the three scales most often mentioned in earlier prospective and retrospective studies of CHD. Further strong evidence for the anxiety hypothesis comes from the prospective Israeli study of MEDALIE *et al.* [1973b] which reports that a three-item anxiety index was prospectively associated (at $p = 0.01$) with the incidence of angina pectoris, with high scorers developing twice the incidence of AP as did low scorers. This scale was not predictive of MI, however.

A confirmatory study by EASTWOOD and TREVELYAN [1971] screened 2,200 English citizens who were on medical practitioners lists. The study administered psychological screening questionnnaires followed by interviews in an effort to identify persons with psychiatric problems. The identified subjects, mostly manifesting chronic mild anxiety and depression were matched with control subjects and both groups were given thorough cardiological examinations. More 'possible and probable CHD' was found in the anxious-depressed group. This CHD excess was significant both for the male and female portions of the matched samples.

Life Dissatisfactions

New evidence has been published that life dissatisfactions serve as a precursor to angina pectoris (AP) and perhaps also to MI. The prospective study by Medalie *et al.* [1973b] showed that problems and conflicts in the areas of finance, family, work, co-workers and superiors were all associated prospectively with development of AP. Each of these areas of satisfaction was tapped by three or four questions and a large number of significant associations with AP emerged. The authors concluded that the intensity of the problem and not its specific content was the critical issue. Men reporting severe problems either with regard to their family or their co-workers incurred about two and a half times the rate of new AP as men reporting no problems in these areas. A combined score for all five problem areas also generated a similar relative risk gradient. These factors were not found associated with risk of new MI in this population.

The matched sample study by Thiel *et al.*]1973] found a sharply decreased sense of enjoyment and increased loneliness in MI patients attributed to the time before the onset of illness. Theorell and Rahe [1972] found post-MI patients in Stockholm to report more work dissatisfaction and less financial dissatisfaction than healthy controls. Other kinds of dissatisfaction did not differ between the two groups in this study. Kavanagh and Shephard [1973] found what they felt was a high frequency of business and social problems in their 102 middle class post-MI patients (no control group).

The findings of increased life problems and dissatisfactions among persons who later develop AP are consistent with the findings regarding anxiety and neuroticism reported earlier. The relation of life dissatisfactions to MI is more equivocal and needs further study using prospective design. The negative findings from the Israeli study of MI, however, make the outlook for positive findings pessimistic. This may be an area in which these two clinical presentations of CHD are sharply different.

Stress and Life Change

One of the chronic life stresses previously reported to be associated with increased risk of CHD is excessive overtime work. THEORELL and RAHE [1972] compared 62 post-MI patients in Stockholm with 109 healthy employees of a municipal agency and found that the MI patients had been doing much more overtime work but had lower responsibility and less supervisory activity than the healthy controls. The difference in the institutional sources from which the two groups came might account for some of these work-related differences, however. Similarly, THIEL *et al.* [1973], reported that 13 of their 50 MI patients had been working more than 70 h/week.

A substantial number of studies using summary measures of life change (particularly the HOLMES and RAHE schedule [1967]) have appeared in the last 4 years. Many of these studies are flawed by lack of adequate comparison groups. Several studies used the CHD patients as their own controls, comparing life change scores in the 6 months preceding infarction with the scores obtained by recall from earlier periods of the patients' lives. A comparison group is necessary in order to rule out the possiblity that the apparent increase in number of life changes for the most recent period is not merely an effect of recent memory being more complete than distant memory.

The following findings have been reported from retrospective studies. Persons experiencing sudden death were reported by next of kin to have experienced a threefold increase in magnitude of life change score from earlier years to the last 6 months of life (no control group) [RAHE and LIND, 1971]. One study of 54 post-infarction patients showed a similar crescendo of life change scores in the 6 months preceding the MI, but only for those patients who had no previous history of CHD. Those with prior heart disease had generally higher life change scores at all times covered by the interview [THEORELL and RAHE, 1971]. Another retrospective study of 30 male post-MI patients showed no such crescendo of life change immediately prior to infarction. There was considerable variability over the several years covered by the recall interview [RAHE and PAASIKIVI, 1971].

A comparable project conducted by the same team in Helsinki showed a rising rate of life change for the 6 months immediately preceding MI (no control group) [RAHE *et al.,* 1973]. The same study showed that interviews with patients' spouses generated similar average life change scores as those with the patients themselves, but the comparison was in terms of group means and not by the more revealing method of a distribution of differences between husband-wife pairs.

The findings thus far generated with regard to a possible association between increased rate of life changes and the timing of MI are by no means conclusive but are such as to warrant careful prospective investigation.

Coronary-Prone Behavior Pattern

Numerous studies published in the last few years have tested further the hypothesis that high risk of CHD occurs in persons having the 'coronary-prone behavior pattern', a style of behavior characterized by striving for achievement, competitiveness, impatience, time-urgency, dedication to vocation or a profession, and excesses of drives and aggression. All but one of the studies reviewed found evidence supporting the association of at least some part of this coronary-prone behavior pattern ('type A') with incidence or prevalence of CHD.

A controlled retrospective study utilized matched groups of MI patients, other hospitalized patients, and healthy community controls to test 10 hypotheses using composite scales of items to assess each major variable [WARDWELL and BAHNSON, 1973]. Only the hypotheses that the type A behavior pattern and somaticizing were particularly characteristic of MI patients were supported at statistically significant levels. WARDWELL and BAHNSON measured the type A behavior pattern with a scale of 17 items administered in a structured interview. THIEL *et al.* [1973] included 6 questions dealing with the behavior pattern in their interviews of MI patients and controls. They did not present group means for the scale as a whole but found that individual questions about excessive drive and rapid body movements significantly discriminated the MI patients and the other four questions had weak trends in the hypothesized direction.

FRIEDMAN *et al.* [1973] conducted a study of cardiac pathology in 64 cases of sudden deaths and 16 deaths from noncardiovascular causes. They interviewed next of kin to ascertain the behavior pattern of the decedents and found a significantly higher percentage of type A persons among those dying of CHD as compared to those with other causes of death.

A number of European studies have tested the relation of various components of the coronary-prone pattern to CHD in retrospective studies. The monograph by MERTENS and SEGERS [1971] presents in its second section a study of 48 CHD patients and 47 somewhat younger fracture patients from the same hospital. The CHD men are more often from professional, white-collar and business occupations whereas the fracture patients are more frequently manual workers and miners. There is a substantial difference in income between the two groups which may overshadow the attempt to relate social behavioral differences to cardiovascular disease to a substantial degree. There were 27 variables which differed significantly between the groups. These relate variously to type A behavior (works longer hours, feels time pressure, seeks responsibility, strong sense of duty), to life dissatisfaction (wants to change job, marital discord), to social and organizational activities and lack of exercise. To the degree that these findings can be accepted as reflecting real differences between CHD and other patients, the data are supportive of the type A, life dissatisfaction and physical exercise hypotheses.

The study of MI patients in Stockholm by THEORELL and RAHE [1972] states that MIs reported more hostility when slowed by others but showed no differences on expressed need to rush against time deadlines.

GANELINA and KRAEVSKIJ [1971] in the Soviet Union compared 30 control patients matched on occupation with 50 males with CHD (39 MI and 11 AP) all of whom were currently experiencing coronary insufficiency. The study was designed with three personality categories in mind. It was found that 76% of CHD patients but only 23% of controls were categorized in a group which sounds very much like the type A, coronary-prone behavior pattern. This group was marked by high scores on strength of will, organizing abilities, ambition and acceleration of rate of work. They were not neurotic but were active, sociable, and held high social ideals. This is clearly concordant with the coronary-prone behavior pattern and with the findings of MERTENS and SEGERS [1971].

An interesting sidelight on the relation of this behavior pattern to coronary disease is revealed in a social-ecologic study by APPELS [1972]. He found high, significant correlations between nationally published mortality rates for arteriosclerotic heart disease (including CHD) and the rank ordering of the prominence of achievement themes in children's storybooks from the same nations as they were quantified by MCCLELLAND and others.

BONAMI and RIME [1972] performed a prospective analysis on responses to the Van Lennep Four Picture Test as these were recorded in personnel files of a large corporation. These projective tests were taken an average of 9.7 years before the emergence of clinical CHD in 32 men. These were compared with the stories given by 40 control subjects well matched on age, education, occupational level, and length of time in the organization. The men who later developed CHD showed a greater need for achievement and greater concentration on their socioprofessional setting at the expense of attention to their family and to recreation. This is an interesting use of personnel records and 'blind' study design to perform a prospective study retrospectively.

The Western Collaborative Group Study was the first prospective study to have included at intake a structured interview specifically designed to measure the coronary-prone behavior pattern. Reports of the incidence of clinical CHD in men previously healthy after 4.5, 6.5, and 8.5 years of surveillance have shown that men judged to possess the coronary-prone behavior pattern (type A) at intake had 1.7–4.5 times the rate of new CHD as men judged to possess the converse, relaxed, easy going pattern, type B. The relative risk ratio observed differs by the age group at intake and the length of follow-up, with younger type A men generating higher relative risk ratios than older men [ROSENMAN *et al.,* 1970, 1971, 1974].

Several studies have also used a self-administered, computer-scored questionnaire for determination of the coronary-prone behavior pattern (the Jenkins Activity Survey). Two studies have reported the association of type A scores derived from this test with prevalence of CHD. In the Western Collaborative Group Study 83 CHD patients scored significantly higher than 524 controls [JENKINS *et al.,* 1971a] and in the study at Bridgeport Connecticut Hospital 48 CHD patients (both men and women) scored significantly higher than 42 patients hospitalized with other diseases [KENIGSBERG *et al.,* 1974]. There is now evidence that Activity Survey scores are also predictive of risk of new CHD. In a prospective study (part of the WCGS) men scoring in the top third of the type A score distribution incurred 1.7 times as much CHD as those scoring in the bottom third or type B end of the distribution [JENKINS *et al.,* 1974]. Type A scores on this test are also associated with increased risk of reinfarction among persons already having CHD. This has been found in two independent samples drawn from the WCGS [JENKINS *et al.,* 1971b].

In two unpublished dissertations using CHD patients from North Carolina and Hawaii, respectively, it was found in both instances that men with CHD had significantly higher mean scores on the type A scale of the Activity Survey than did comparison groups without disease [STOKOLS, 1973; COHEN, 1974].

The one study which found negative evidence concerning the type A behavior pattern was the historical prospective analysis of the Kaiser-Permanente data [FRIEDMAN *et al.,* 1974]. A 155-item true-false inventory (which dealt largely with interpersonal problems and neurotic symptoms) had been administered to thousands of health plan subscribers in earlier years. Researchers familiar with the coronary-prone pattern were asked to select those items from this pool which would be characteristic of type A and type B respondents. Two type A experts reported problems in use of these questions to identify type A persons but nevertheless presented lists of items which had considerable overlap. Neither of the sets of items selected (nor the common items selected by both raters) were predictive of the persons who later developed MI in this study group. It should be pointed out that in contrast to most other studies reported in this section, this one included both men and women over a wide age range including persons over 70 years of age.

In summary, much evidence has been published by a number of research teams which collectively gives strong added support to the hypothesis that the coronary-prone behavior pattern, type A, is associated retrospectively and prospectively both with risk of new CHD in healthy persons and risk of reinfarction in persons already having CHD. The number of independent studies reporting consistent findings is greater for the type A behavior pattern than for any of the other major categories of psychosocial variables.

Other Traits and Defenses

Various other personality traits, psychological defenses and response sets have been implicated from time to time as being associated with risk of CHD. Important among these is the tendency to exaggerated unsophisticated defenses such as denial. In addition to earlier work by HACKETT and CASSEM [1969] and VAN DER VALK and GROEN [1967], further support for the prominence of denial in CHD patients is offered by the study of CROOG *et al.* [1971] which found that among 345 survivors of MI, 20% denied that they even had had a heart attack within 3 weeks of the event. Denial was characteristic of many aspects of the lives of these patients. They denied having unfavorable traits, having a family history of heart disease, and denied having certain physical symptoms. The pattern persisted over the 1-year follow-up period, thus giving the appearance of an enduring trait. In CROOG'S sample this massive denial was more common in Jewish and Italian patients than in Irish and English patients. No comparison groups without CHD were available to this study.

Indirect support for the denial hypothesis comes from two additional studies. THOMAS and GREENSTREET [1973] in their prospective study of medical students found that the eight who later developed acute MI gave the fewest Rorschach responses on the average and also reported greatest closeness to parents. These observations are suggestive of great defensiveness, constriction of imagery and fear of independent expression. BONAMI and RIME [1972] in a prospective study previously described found that the projective test responses given by men who later developed CHD were more ambivalent, more tightly structured, and more restricted in fantasy. This does not echo the theme of denial, but certainly is in keeping with a more general pattern of exaggerated defenses.

Studies in the Netherlands and the US point to the possibility of a tendency for MI patients to endorse extreme categories of scaled multiple choice items. This seems to be a response set independent of the content of the items. VAN DIJL and OLTHUIS [1970] report a retrospective study of 123 MI patients and 482 healthy controls. Their questionnaire consisted of 69 scaled items, each having six categories for possible response, similar to a semantic differential scale. On many scales the infarct patients showed a preference for extreme responses in both directions, whereas the control patients distributed their responses more in a bell-shaped curve. The retrospective matched sample study by THIEL *et al.* [1973] found a tendency for MI patients to exhibit extreme behaviors with regard to sports participation (either doing nothing or participating in many sports). A sizable minority also reported extremes in fluid consumption, work hours, and smoking. These responses did not occur as frequently among controls. The findings from these two studies are seen as a confirmation of the position of VAN DER VALK and GROEN [1967] who claim that a major feature of MI patients is an exaggeration of otherwise normal behaviors of today's Western culture.

The role of the central nervous system in the etiology of CHD is given further support by the predictive value of a very different type of behavioral test: the rise in blood pressure during the cold pressor test. In this test the subject inserts his hand and forearm into a bucket of ice water. Certain physiologic changes are then measured. KEYS *et al.* [1971] used this procedure in a longitudinal study of 279 men followed for 20 years. Among the 20 variables measured, rise in diastolic blood pressure during the cold pressor test was the strongest single predictor of subsequent CHD, followed closely by serum cholesterol and systolic blood pressure. THOMAS and GREENSTREET [1973] report a longitudinal study of 1,030 white male medical students. Due to the young age of their study group only 8 had developed MI at the time of their 1973 report. Compared to groups of various sizes developing other diseases and the large remnant remaining well, these future MI cases showed at initial exam the highest rise in systolic blood pressure in response to the cold pressor test. The findings from these two independent studies should provoke further use of this test and other techniques for estimating the reactivity of the physiological system to a standard challenge in future studies of CHD risk.

Conclusion

This paper has attempted to sketch a comprehensive picture of the status in mid-1974 of psychosomatically-oriented field studies of atherosclerotic and coronary heart disease. Several review articles are cited which give broad coverage to research on this topic published before 1970. Building upon this foundation, this paper attempts to summarize progress by research teams in many countries in specifying the nature of the association between CHD and such categories of precursors as sociologic indexes, social mobility and status incongruity, anxiety and neuroticism, life dissatisfations, stress and life change, the coronary-prone behavior pattern, and other traits and defenses. Several epidemiological studies which considered myocardial infarction and angina pectoris separately have found that these two presentations of CHD have different psychosocial precursors.

It is this reviewer's belief that the primary research need in this area is not for further exploratory studies, but rather for carefully designed hypothesis-testing studies which will serve to sort out and clarify the exciting but disorganized array of positive findings already reported (and in many cases replicated) in the scientific literature. This can best be done in large-scale prospective studies of CHD incidence which pay careful attention both to measurement of the psychosocial variables and to ascertainment of clinical diagnosis by standard criteria. Another promising direction is the study of psychosocial variables in connection with distinct pathogenetic processes of the cardiovascular system. This category of studies would rely on such methods as coronary angiography, measures of sequential changes in hemodynamics and oxygen uptake of the myocardium, studies of blood clotting mechanisms and of alterations in electrical conductivity of the heart muscle.

One thing is certain: psychological and social variables and various aspects of behavioral style are clearly associated with the risk of developing arteriosclerotic and coronary heart disease. It would seem, but with less certainty, that the psychosocial risk factors operate through mechanisms largely independent of the more traditional CHD risk factors, such as elevated blood pressure, serum cholesterol, cigarette smoking, and obesity. It must be remembered in addition that these latter 'biological risk factors' are largely the product of human behavior and the means for their control is through altering habits of living. Thus, both the understanding and modification of the traditional risk factors and of the promising new psychosocial risk factors are challenges which fall primarily into the realm of psychosomatic medicine and the behavioral sciences.

References

APPELS, A.: Het hartinfarct een cultuurziekte? Tijdschr. soc. Geneesk. *50:* 446–448 (1972).

BONAMI, M. and RIME, B.: A study of the personality of pre-coronaries by standardized analysis of thematic projective data. J. psychosom. Res. *16:* 103–113 (1972).

CASSEL, J.C.; HEYDEN, S.; BARTEL, A.G., *et al.:* Incidence of coronary heart disease by ethnic group, social class, and sex. Archs. intern. Med. *128:* 901–906 (1971).

CHRISTIAN, P.: Interdependenz von Umwelt und Person am Beispiel des Herzinfarktes. Psychother. Psychosom. *16:* 210–223 (1968).

COHEN, J.B.: Sociocultural change and behavior patterns in disease etiology: an epidemiologic study of coronary disease among Japanese Americans; Ph.D. Dissertation in Epidemiology, School of Public Health, University of California at Berkeley (1974).

COMSTOCK, G.W. and PARTRIDGE, K.B.: Church attendance and health. J. chron. Dis. *25:* 665 672 (1972).

CROOG, S.H. and LEVINE, S.: Social status and subjective perceptions of 250 men after myocardial infarction. Publ. Hlth Rep. Wash. *84:* 989–997 (1969).

CROOG, S.H.; SHAPIRO, D.S., and LEVINE, S.: Denial among male heart patients. An empirical study. Psychosom. Med. *33:* 385–397 (1971).

EASTWOOD, M.R. and TREVELYAN, H.: Stress and coronary heart disease. J. psychosom. Res. *15:* 289–292 (1971).

FRIEDMAN, G.D.; URY, H.K.; KLATSKY, A.L., and SIEGELAUB, M.S.: A psychological questionnaire predictive of myocardial infarction. Psychosom. Med. *36:* 327–343 (1974).

FRIEDMAN, M.; MANWARING, J.H.; ROSENMAN, R.H., *et al.:* Instantaneous and sudden death: clinical and pathological differentiation in coronary artery disease. J. Am. med. Ass. *225:* 1319–1328 (1973).

GANELINA, I.E. and KRAEVSKIJ, J.M.: Premorbid personality traits in patients with cardiac ischaemia. Cardiologia, Moscow *2:* 40–45 (1971).

GARCIA-PALMIERI, M.; COSTAS, R.; GORDON, T., *et al.:* Differences in coronary heart disease in Honolulu, Puerto Rico and Framingham. Paper presented at 45th Scientific Session of American Heart Ass., Dallas 1972.

GREENE, W.A.; GOLDSTEIN, S., and MOSS, A.J.: Psychosocial aspects of sudden death. Archs intern. Med. *129:* 725–731 (1972).

HACKETT, T.P. and CASSEM, N.H.: Factors contributing to delay in responding to the signs and symptoms of acute myocardial infarction. Am. J. Cardiol. *24:* 651–658 (1969).

HOLMES, T.H. and RAHE, R.H.: The social readjustment rating scale. J. psychosom. Res. *11:* 213–218 (1967).

JENKINS, C.D.: Psychologic and social precursors of coronary disease. New Engl. J. Med. *284:* 244–255, 307–317 (1971).

JENKINS, C.D.; ROSENMAN, R.H., and ZYZANSKI, S.J.: Prediction of clinical coronary heart disease by a test for the coronary-porone behavior pattern. New Engl. J. Med. *290:* 1271–1275 (1974).

JENKINS, C.D.; ZYZANSKI, S.J., and ROSENMAN, R.H.: Progress toward validation of a computer-scored test for the type A coronary-prone behavior pattern. Psychosom. Med. *33:* 193–202 (1971a).

JENKINS, C.D.; ZYZANSKI, S.J.; ROSENMAN, R.H., and CLEVELAND, G.L.: Association of coronary-prone behavior scores with recurrence of coronary heart disease. J. chron. Dis. *24:* 601–611 (1971b).

KAPLAN, B.H.; CASSEL, J.C.; TYROLER, H.A., *et al.:* Occupational mobility and coronary heart disease. Archs. intern. Med. *128:* 938–942 (1971).

KAVANAGH, T. and SHEPHARD, R.J.: The immediate antecedents of myocardial infarction in active men. Can. med. Ass. J. *109:* 19–22 (1973).

KENIGSBERG, D.; ZYZANSKI, S.J.; JENKINS, C.D.; WARDWELL, W.I., and LICCIARDELLO, A.T.: The coronary-prone behavior pattern in hospitalized patients with and without coronary heart disease. Psychosom. Med. *36:* 344–351 (1974).

KEYS, A.: Coronary heart disease in seven countries. Circulation *41:* suppl. 1, pp. 1–211 (1970).

KEYS, A.; ARAVANIS, C.; BLACKBURN, H., *et al.:* Probability of middle-aged men developing coronary heart disease in five years. Circulation *45:* 815–828 (1972).

KEYS, A.; TAYLOR, H.L.; BLACKBURN, H., *et al.:* Mortality and coronary heart disease among men studied for 23 years. Archs. intern. Med. *128:* 201–214 (1071).

LEHR, I.; MESSINGER, H.B., and ROSENMAN, R.H.: A sociobiological approach to the study of coronary heart disease. J. chron. Dis. *26:* 13–30 (1973).

MAI, F.M.M.: Personality and stress in coronary heart disease. J. psychosom. Res. *12:* 275–287 (1968).

MAYOU, R.: The patient with angina. Symptoms and disability. Postgrad. med. J. *49:* 250–254 (1973).

MCDONOUGH, J.R.; HAMES, C.G.; STULB, S.C., *et al.:* Coronary heart disease among Negroes and Whites in Evans County, Georgia. J. chron. Dis. *18:* 443–468 (1965).

MEDALIE, J.H.; KAHN, M.A.; NEUFELD, H.N., *et al.:* Myocardial infarction over a five year period. I. prevalence, incidence and mortality experience. J. chron. Dis. *26:* 63–48 (1973a).

MEDALIE, J.H.; SNYDER, M.; GROEN, J.J., *et al.:* Angina pectoris among 10,000 men: five year incidence and univariate analysis. Am. J. Med. *55:* 583–594 (1973b).

MERTENS, C. et SEGERS, M.J.: L'influence des facteurs psychologiques dans la genèse des affections coronariennes. Bull. Acad. r. Méd. Belg. *11:* 155–221 (1971).

RAHE, R.H. and LIND, E.: Psychosocial factors and sudden cardiac death: a pilot study. J. psychosom. Res. *15:* 19–24 (1971).

RAHE, R.H. and PAASIKIVI, J.: Psychosocial factors and myocardial infarction. II. An outpatients study in Sweden. J. psychosom. Res. *15:* 33–39 (1971).

RAHE, R.H.; ROMO, M.; BENNETT, L., and SILTANEN, P.: Subjects' recent life changes and myocardial infarction in Helsinki. Manuscript duplicated by US Navy Medical Neuropsychiatric Research Unit. San Diego (1973).

ROSENMAN, R.H.: Assessing the risk associated with behavior patterns. J. med. Ass. Georgia 31–34 (February 1971).

ROSENMAN, R.H.; FRIEDMAN, M.; STRAUS, R., *et al.*: Coronary heart disease in the Western Collaborative Group Study: a follow-up experience of 4½ years. J. chron. Dis. *23:* 173–190 (1970).

ROSENMAN, R.H.; JENKINS, C.D.; BRAND, R.J., *et al.*: Coronary heart disease in the Western Collaborative Group Study: final follow-up experience of 8½ years. J. Am. med. Ass. (in press, 1974).

RUSKIN, H.D.; STEIN, L.L.; SHELSKY, I.M., *et al.*: MMPI comparison between patients with coronary heart disease and their spouses together with other demographic data. Scand. J. Rehab. Med. *23:* 99–104 (1970).

SIGURJONSSON, J.: Occupational variations in mortality from ischemic heart disease. J. Am. Geriat. Soc. *19:* 34–40 (1971).

STOKOLS, J.J.: Life dissatisfaction as a risk factor in coronary heart disease; Ph.D. Dissertation in Psychology, University of North Carolina at Chapel Hill (1973).

SYME, S.L.; HYMAN, M.M., and ENTERLINE, P.E.: Cultural mobility and the occurrence of coronary heart disease. J. Hlth hum. Behav. *6:* 178–189 (1965).

THEORELL, T. and RAHE, R.H.: Psychosocial factors and myocardial infarction. I. An inpatient study in Sweden. J. psychsom. Res. *15:* 25–31 (1971).

THEORELL, T. and RAHE, R.H.: Behavior and life satisfactions characteristics of Swedish subjects with myocardial infarction. J. chron. Dis. *25:* 139–147 (1972).

THIEL, H.G.; PARKER, D., and BRUCE, T.A.: Stress factors and the risk of myocardial infarction. J. psychosom. Res. *17:* 43–57 (1973).

THOMAS, C.B. and GREENSTREET, R.L.: Psychobiological characteristics in youth as predictors of five disease states: suicide, mental illness, hypertension, coronary heart disease and tumor. Johns Hopkins med. J. *132:* 16–43 (1973).

VAN DER VALK, J.M. and GROEN, J.J.: Personality structure and conflict situation in patients with myocardial infarction. J. psychosom. Res. *11:* 41–46 (1967).

VAN DIJL, H. and OLTHUIS, F.H.: Some test behavior differences between healthy men and male myocardial infarction patients. Psychother. Psychosom. *18:* 286–293 (1970).

WARDWELL, W.I. and BAHNSON, C.B.: Behavioral variables and myocardial infarction in the Southeastern Connecticut Heart Study. J. chron. Dis. *26:* 447–461 (1973).

WEISS, N.S.: Marital status and risk factors for coronary heart diease. The United States Health Examination Survey of adults. Br. J. Prev. Soc. Med. *27:* 41–43 (1973).

WILLIAMS, A.O.: Coronary atherosclerosis in Nigeria. Br. Heart J. *33:* 95–100 (1971).

WILLIAMS, C.A.: The relationship of occupational change to blood pressure, serum cholesterol, a specific overt behavior pattern and coronary heart disease; Dissertation, Department of Epidemiology, University of North Carolina (1968).

C. DAVID JENKINS, Ph.D., Director, Department of Behavioral Epidemiology, Boston University School of Medicine, *Boston, MA 02118* (USA)

Adv. psychosom. Med., vol. 9, pp. 20–37 (Karger, Basel 1977)

Rapid Sociocultural Change and High Blood Pressure

A.M. OSTFELD and D.A. D'ATRI

Department of Epidemiology and Public Health, Yale University School of Medicine, New Haven, Conn.

In the past 20 years, most of the work on the psychosocial epidemiology of high blood pressure has focused on a single hypothesis, sometimes vaguely, sometimes precisely formulated. In its simplest terms, the hypothesis is that rapid sociocultural changes leads to psychological stress and subsequently to high blood pressure. Stable, traditional societies will exhibit little or no high blood pressure and little or no rise in blood pressure with age. In societies undergoing rapid transition, the opposite will be noted. This review is concerned with the two decades of research bearing on the hypothesis. Some work of merit not dealing directly with this hypothesis is not reviewed.

At a conference in 1964, OSTFELD and SHEKELLE [1] reviewed the literature on the psychosocial epidemiology of primary hypertension. This included the two acute epidemics of high blood pressure in Texas City and near El Alamein, both, regrettably epidemics of rather uncertain duration [2,3]. Eight studies published by then showed differences in the prevalence of high blood pressure, in frequency distributions of blood pressure, and in the possible rate of rise of pressure with age in populations with different degrees of urbanization and industrialization [4–11]. The authors noted that their studies were cross-sectional, not longitudinal, and that differences in genetic endowment, diet, body bulk and prevalence of infection in the groups studied obscured the clear determination of the relevance of cultural change and psychosocial stress to the differences in blood pressure characteristics.

OSTFELD and SHEKELLE [1] wrote, 'a succession of workers, the recent ones being epidemiologists, rediscover serially that blood pressure responds with surprising magnitude to emotion-provoking stimuli. Each speculates about the meaning of this for high blood pressure and no one seems to have been able to get beyond this point [11]. In an effort to proceed further with understanding these relationships, they presented two hypotheses.

(1) Life situations that evoke pressor responses are characterized by uncertainty, the possibility of bodily or psychological harm, the inappropriateness of running or fighting, and the need to maintain a vigilant mental attitude until the situation is clarified or ended.

(2) The breakdown of traditional, well-defined societies leads to conflict about social roles and to more of those ambiguous, threatening life situations that raise blood pressure.

LOVELL, at the same conference, reviewed his own experience in the Fiji and Gilbert Islands [4, 12], and the data from a wide variety of populations including Chinese [13, 14], American Indian [15, 16], Australoid [17, 18], Indo-Malay [19, 20], Bushmen [7], Negroid [21, 22], Micronesian [6, 23], Polynesian [24, 25], Melanesian [4, 6, 26, 27], and Europeans in Europe and the United States [28–31]. He concluded that among rural young men, there was a consistent correlation between measures of body bulk and blood pressures, consistent across ethnic and racial lines. The same correlation was less evident for older persons of both sexes. In the Southwest Pacific, most groups studied did not show an increase in systolic pressure with increasing age, a correlation characteristic of those of European stock. In some cases, older people had lower pressures, than younger people in the Southwest Pacific.

At the same conference, SHAPER [32] reported on 3 nomadic pastoral tribes in Northern Kenya, noting that no increase in blood pressure with increasing age was evident. He measured weight [3], skinfold thickness, ponderal index and blood pressure among a group of 52 traditional warrior tribesmen and 74 similar men who had served a few months to 11 years in the army. The army men measured higher on every variable assessed including blood pressure and ate a diet of about 50% carbohydrates, whereas the nomadic tribesmen consumed fat and protein almost exclusively. The data were cross-sectional.

In only three of all these studies were the populations defined, *Shaper's* [32] village study, and MADDOCKS' [5, 6] data in the Fiji and Gilbert Islands. The rest were 'chunk samples' or 'samples of convenience'.

There were, at that time, at least two methods of examining the hypothesis that stable, traditional societies exhibit lower pressures and smaller rates of rise of pressures with age than societies in a state of transition. One was to examine two or more genetically related groups among whom societal patterns, but little else affecting blood pressure, varied; that is, the cross-sectional approach. The other was to identify a stable, traditional society, learn to understand its language and its organization and follow the group with serial blood pressure determinations over as long as two decades while the anticipated cultural and social change occurred; the longitudinal approach.

It was already apparent, at the meeting at which these hypotheses were presented[1] and discussed that there would be trouble in implementing them. An internist said of this kind of research 'one way is to take your blood pressure, log a lot of sociological variables, put them into a computer and something is bound to correlate with something else'. Another internist complained, 'in some of the groups we have worked amongst, it has taken an anthropologist living with the tribe 3 or 4 years not only to learn the language but become accepted within the group. Even then, the responses of that group to him were still, of course, not the responses they would have to each other. He was a foreign element in a rigid society'. Because there were only 2 social scientists at the meeting of 54 investigators, their comments about the failures of internist-epidemiologists were more muted. That should not be taken to mean that the internists' observations on social and cultural data were detailed, precise, or well organized. They were not. The social scientists had much to criticize but evidentally decided to withhold their fire. Consider this bit of ammunition provided by an internist that the social scientists did not use. In trying to explain why a colleague's blood pressure measurements were lower than those made in the same group a couple of years earlier, he replied, 'I don't know why these pressures are higher than Maddocks' pressures in the same tribal area. I wonder if the reason is that Whyte was one of the first surveyors in this part of New Guinea visiting with a patrol officer perhaps concerned with such things as collecting taxes. Also during his survey, blood was taken for cholesterol. ... Dr. Ian Maddocks who has done a lot of the field work on this area thinks it may make a considerable difference if you arrive with a patrol officer or if you go along knowing the people and are able to sit down and chat quietly with them, as he can do'.

Two papers stand out among this earlier work. NORMAN-TAYLOR and REES [27] studied three communities in the New Hebrides. The participation rates in the communities were provided and ranged from 60 to 80% of the entire communities. The criteria for blood pressure measurements were clear and the difficulties in recognizing age were acknowledged. Weights and

1 The meeting was held in 1964 and the book based on it published in 1967.

heights were not recorded but no obesity was grossly apparent. Two of the communities were described as being 'virtually untouched by civilization' and in the third, that consisted of suburbs of the administrative capital of New Hebrides there was already substantial urbanization and European influence. In the latter most of the inhabitants were wage earners in the towns and ate a diet like that of the local Europeans. The mean systolic and diastolic blood pressures of all three communities, together numbering 713, did not differ from one another and showed no appreciable rise with age. Most of the blood pressures were measured by a single investigator.

The best of the early work, although often cited, is worth reciting. SCOTCH [10, 11] conducted field work in two Zulu communities in South Africa in 1958/59, one rural native reserve and another in an urban location outside Durban. Interviews were conducted with systematic random samples of 548 persons in the rural area and 505 in the urban. Blood pressures assessed in a standard manner, age, weight, height, and questions about education, health, income, religion, and daily behavior comprised the variables of concern. The mean blood pressures of the urban Zulu were substantially higher than those in the rural preserve. Age and obesity showed the usual correlation with blood pressure. In the urban community, those with higher pressures were the ones who maintained traditional cultural practices. SCOTCH considered that rapid culture change may lead to social and psychological stress and then to hypertension and called for framing more specific hypotheses relating cultural change to high blood pressure. SCOTCH, an anthropologist, had good medical, epidemiological and biostatistical consultants. He showed the way in 1958/59 and most others did not follow.

The crucial point in presenting these two best of the earlier papers is to show that one did not support the hypotheses relating high blood pressure and rise in pressure with age to sociocultural change and the other provided no ringing confirmation of it.

HENRY and CASSEL [33] laid most of the published studies on psychosocial factors in essential hypertension on the procrustean bed of their hypothesis (the sociocultural change hypothesis) and made them fit. When Americans moving to China in the 1920s had a probable decline in blood pressure [34], the hypothesis was not violated because – in the view of HENRY and CASSEL – the American immigrants saw the light of the calm Chinese order of things and their jobs as missionary hospital staff 'decreased the anxiety level' and 'increased their self-esteem'. Maybe so but where are the data? When the only longitudinal blood pressure data in 25 studies cited, the 24-year follow-up of 1,000 US Naval aviators [35], showed no rise in mean blood pressure with age, this was attributed to the notion that they were 'only men thoroughly adapted from youth to the demands of a technological society'. The facts that they were born about 1920, knew the great depression, went into the military, fought in the war, returned to civilian life or to the peacetime navy, sometimes moved permanently to other countries, both industrialized and developing, are all neglected in a consideration of the data. Are these evidence of cultural and social change or not? Certainly they ought not to be forgotten in considering the hypothesis.

It is worth noting that those aviators whose pressures did rise with age were those who gained weight and had one or more parents die early. Weight gain had a more important effect than the heredo-familial factor.

In the remainder of the work reviewed by HENRY and CASSEL, those papers not cited earlier in the present report did in general lend some support to the hypothesis. Data from the Guatemalan highlands [36], urban Chinese living in Taiwan [37], the disintegrating Washo tribe forced to leave its ancestral homeland and way of life and live in squatter's shacks around Carson City [38], Japanese farmers [39], and Indian villagers [20] all exhibited some evidence that rapid cultural and social change leading to conflict are correlated positively with blood pressure levels and possibly with higher rates of rise of pressure with age.

The more recent work, not summarized elsewhere deserves a less telegraphic review. STROTZ and SHORR [40] analyzed data obtained from the outpatient records of 61% (4,400) of the 7,281 Papago Indians who used the Indian Health Service Outpatient Department from 1963 to 1969. They observed a 20% prevalence of blood pressures equalling or exceeding 160/95, a proportion that did not increase with age although mean pressures increased with age. Less than a quarter of the tribe followed the traditional Indian way. The prevalence of diabetes was 16% (diagnosed by a physician) and 43% of the diabetics but only 15% of the non-diabetics were hypertensive. This association strongly implicates obesity as the underlying determinant of the hypertension and diabetes. Although weights were not presented, the authors described the major changes in diet from meat to carbohydrates after world war II. Regrettably blood pressures for those following and not following the traditional Indian way are not presented separately.

A paper by TENBRINCK [41] typifies material that is still being published but is lacking in scientific value. The blood pressures of 106 Apaches on the Whiteriver Reservation, Arizona; some, the parents of children examined at the reservation medical facility, some hospital employees, and some, visitors who became interested in the study, were recorded and compared with an equally carefully drawn sample of Shepibo Indians in Brazil obtained earlier by the same author. We are informed that the Shepibo and Apache came from different stocks, live in different climates but that 'both live relatively simply in undeveloped communities'. This is followed by the astounding revelation that obesity and heart disease attack some Apaches early while other survive into old age. Finally, the data from the Apache are compared with those from the Build and Blood Pressure Study of the Society of Actuaries, and it is noted that the Apache pressures are lower.

In a superior study, TSENG [42] surveyed the blood pressures of two neighboring populations, one agricultural and one fishing, in southwest Taiwan. 70% of the farming population over age 15 and 62% of the fishing population cooperated in the survey. For persons over 30, the response rates were 81 and 76%, respectively. 15 physicians measured the pressures in a standard manner. The prevalence of pressures over 160/95 was nearly twice as high in the fishing communitites as among the agricultural ones. The fishermen's pressures were higher than those recorded in another survey in Taipei and higher than the US National Health Survey data. Pressures rose with age in both groups. Both populations have maintained their traditional diet, habits, customs, culture and religion for over 300 years, characteristics which have not been changed by the Chinese occupation or the rising tide of westernization. The farmers are rural and the fishermen live in overcrowded communities. Perhaps the crowded circumstances among the fishermen are related to the higher prevalence of high blood pressure. The complex relationship between crowding and blood pressure, a relationship not further considered in this chapter, has recently been examined by D'ATRI and OSTFELD [43].

LANGFORD *et al.* [44] studied 98% of the black female high school students, 2,600 persons, in Jackson, Mississippi and surrounding rural Hinds County. Blood pressures were measured both with a London School of Tropical Medicine and Hygiene manometer and then with a standard manometer. Height, weight, arm circumference, skinfold thickness, and pulse rate were also determined. Black nurses in black schools checked the effect of white and black visitors on blood pressure. Pressures were significantly higher in rural Hinds County than in Jackson, and in Jackson there was an inverse correlation between socioeconomic status and pressures. The socioeconomic status was estimated by housing data using as criteria the proportion of 'sound' housing units, proportion of housing units having 1 person per room or more and average owner value or rental value of housing units for each block in Jackson. Socioeconomic status was not determined in the rural area because of lack of sound data. The same pattern of higher pressures in the country and of a socioeconomic gradient in the city was found in black boys as well as in white girls and white boys later surveyed with the same discipline and high quality.

These authors are not the only ones to record high blood pressure in rural than in urban area. MIALL and COCHRANE [45] in Jamaica found that rural women had higher pressures than urban women. REID *et al.* [46] noted higher pressures among rural mail carriers than mail carriers in London. And the national Health Survey reported that blood pressures were higher in rural than in urban Americans [47]. Without more data, no one could argue seriously that rural means stable and traditional and that urban means rapidly changing, but it is even less defensible to argue that the reverse is true.

There is no question that the southeastern US has higher blood pressures and higher stroke mortality than any other part of the country [29, 44, 48–52]. The high death rates from hypertension in the south may be in part a reflection of low income and a rural environment. Yet in some ways the south was until recently, culturally and socially one of the more stable parts of the United States. While black migration was to the urban north whites stayed in their own or neighboring states even when they moved [52–57]. Agriculture was predominant, large cities were few and recent European immigration small and largely limited to New Orleans and East Central Texas. The traditions of caste, class, and behavior were strong. No facile explanations cover these relationships.

JORGENSON *et al.* [58], studied the Amish Community of Somerset County, Pennsylvania and Garrett County, Maryland. This is an endogamous population separated from the rest of the community for religious reasons. Sharing common ancestors, the group exhibits cultural heterogeneity. There are four degrees of compliance with contemporary American lifeways. 56% of the total Amish community or a total of 780 subjects participated. In addition to careful standard assessments of blood pressure, weight, height, medical history, and membership in a specific subgroup within the Amish were recorded. Systolic but not diastolic pressures exhibited a clear upward trend with decreasing cultural conservatism and there was only a small increase with increasing age in any of the subgroups, except that the Old Order Amish, the most conservative of all the groups, showed even less rise of pressure with age than the Beachy Amish, the conservative Mennonites and the Mennonites, three subgroups with increasing liberality in the order named.

JOHNSON [59] carried out a meritorious blood pressure survey in a crowded urban West African population in Lagos. The Department of Community

Health of the Lagos University College of Medicine has maintained 30 survey sample blocks chosen on a random systematic basis as a community laboratory. The areas of the study were chosen at random from these survey blocks. Apparently the participation rate was near 100% and all data were collected in homes by the author. Standard blood pressures, age, marital status, occupation, education and household relationships were recorded. The mean blood pressures were generally higher and arterial hypertension more prevalent than in some white populations in the United States [60], Norway [61] and in England [62]. The Lagos readings were also lower than those recorded by COMSTOCK among blacks in Muscogee County, Georgia [51] and very close to those reported by SCOTCH [11] in the Zulu. The Lagos pressures, systolic and diastolic, rose progressively with age, in parallel with the Bergen data of BOE *et al.* [61], the Tecumseh data [63] and HAMILTON's British observations [62].

PRIOR *et al.* [64, 65] have carried out a unique and promising series of investigations in the Southwest Pacific. Ruatahuna, Tikitiki and Rotorua, three New Zealand Maori communities whose lifeways ranged from traditional to Europeanized, were surveyed in a standard manner with excellent response rates. Blood pressures did not differ in the three groups. Pressures in the traditional community did not differ from those in the westernized groups, although the latter exhibited a rise with age and the former did not. As with blood pressures, heights, weights and skinfold thicknesses were essentially the same in the three groups.

In the Cook Islands, PRIOR *et al.* [64] also studied two communities; Pukapuka, isolated and traditional, and Rarotonga, largely Europeanized. The Rarotongans had higher blood pressures at all ages and a greater rise in pressures with age. They were also taller and heavier. The Rarotongan women who are described as being unusually obese had a steep rise in pressure with age; much more so than the men.

In an intriguing study PRIOR [65] compared people who subsequently migrated with those who stayed at home on the Tokelau Islands. The response rates were exceptionally high and standard methods of measurement were employed. The study had the further advantage that the demography and social anthropology of the islanders had been surveyed earlier. In the entire population, weight, skinfold thickness and blood pressures rose with increasing age. Both pre-migrants and non-migrants showed a moderate increase in pressure with age. The younger male pre-migrants – but not women or older men – were taller, heavier, had higher pressures and urinary sodium excretions that their non-migrating counterparts. The authors speculate that younger, more athletic males migrate actively and that the women and older men acquiesce in their decision. PRIOR cautions that much of the difference between pre-migrant and non-migrant young men is attributable to a relatively small group of tall heavy pre-migrants with fairly high blood pressures. A longitudinal study of these people is promised and its results ought to prove illuminating.

FLOREY and CUADRADO [66] had a unique opportunity to learn something about blood pressure and took full advantage of it. The Cape Verde Islands in the North Atlantic have been inhabited by a mixed African and Portuguese population which began to settle in New England in moderate numbers by 1924. In the Cape Verdes, a single island, Sao Nicolau, was chosen for study because preliminary inquiry among US dwellers of Cape Verdean descent indicated that the island was the original home named most often by New England Cape Verdeans. In Sao Nicolau, a two-stage sampling procedure was followed, a probability sampling of the villages followed by quota sampling within villages. In the US the entire Cape Verdean community of Waterbury, Connecticut was enumerated. 80% of all those with two Verdean parents participated in the study. About 110 volunteers from New Bedford, Massachusetts shown to be homogeneous with the Waterbury group completed the US sample. The Sao Nicolau group studied numbered 491, with a completion rate of about 68%. Blood pressure, arm girth, age, sex, height, and weight were recorded in a standard manner. ABO blood group studies confirmed the ethnic homogeneity in Sao Nicolau and in New Bedford. The New England men had higher pressures for each age and a great rate of rise with age than the Cape Verdeans. The pressure for women did not differ in either respect. The correlations of systolic and diastolic pressures with weight for men and women, New Englanders and Cape Verdeans, ranged from 0.216 to 0.581. The New Englanders were significantly heavier in both sexes and all age groups. Most important of all, when appropriate mathematical adjustments of the regression of blood pressure were made to take weight into account, the pressure differences between the two populations disappeared. In other words, if weight could have been held constant, the blood pressures of the New Englanders would be expected to be the same as those of the Islanders.

The last study to be reviewed is the Framingham inquiry; in particular, the evidence relating obesity to blood pressure and hypertension [67]. The population consisted of 5,127 men and women aged 30–62 years and followed for over 12 years at the time of the publication reviewed here. All subjects, in addition to the well-known measurements of the study, were assigned a relative weight based on average population weights which were height and sex specific. Skinfold thicknesses were also taken into account. Overweight was a powerful predictor of hypertension; the greater the obesity, the larger the subsequent increase in blood pressure. Moreover, the pressures rose and fell with weight over the 12 years of observation. Pressures were measured on the forearm as well as the upper arm to minimize the contribution of arm girth as opposed to weight. But obese subjects of equal relative weight had similar blood pressures irrespective of arm girth and the independent effect of arm girth on pressure was not significant.

The relationship between overweight and high blood pressure in cross-sectional studies is one of the most consistent of all physiological relationships in man [68–70]. Hypertensives have been shown to be heavier than those without elevated pressures [71, 72]. The converse has also been shown to be true [73]. Normotensive obese subjects have been demonstrated to develop more hypertension while under medical observation than those who are not obese [74]. Most convincing of all, blood pressures have been shown to increase with weight and to decrease with spontaneous or prescribed weight reduction [75]. The Framingham study strongly supports these observations [76]. We will come back to the relationship between weight and blood pressure a little later.

All but a handful of the numerous studies cited here are guilty of several of the following methodological failures or oversights.

(1) The variables of cultural change, social change, and psychosocial stresses are still not defined precisely, not assessed in a standard way or not described in enough detail to permit replication.

(2) The blood pressures are not recorded in a standard manner.

(3) The social and cultural assessments are not made in ignorance of what the blood pressure readings are, and vice versa.

(4) Social scientists are still relatively uninvolved. The data of moment are usually brief general qualitative descriptions by physicians, without discipline or standard methods.

(5) The samples are usually 'chunk' or 'convenience' samples, which means anybody around who lets his blood pressure be taken.

(6) Only one new longitudinal study of blood pressure and sociocultural change has been undertaken to test the hypothesis posed here.

(7) Age is less accurately known in some societies than in others, and its correlation with blood pressure in some settings is uncertain. In some areas there were no vital statistics, no birth certificates, no calendars and no recorded time.

What does it all mean that blood pressures rise with age in some settings and not in others?

Since it is unlikely that higher pressures lead to increasing chronological age, an association between blood pressure and age is more likely to mean that pressure increases because of age rather than the other way round. But the lack of an association between age and blood pressure can also mean that elevated blood pressures are rapidly lethal in that group (a prospective study would show this), or that a systematic bias occurred in which young people with higher pressures and old people with low pressures tended to get into the survey, or that the inception of cultural and social change had greater pressor effects in the young than in the old or induced overweight more rapidly in the young than in the old. Or that young people in some groups have larger arms. Or even that the observers measured pressures in such a way as to confirm their expectations of no rise or a rise with age.

The problem is compounded by the fact that in longitudinal studies, blood pressures are higher on the initial examination than they are 3–5 years later [35, 76, 77]. Cross-sectional blood pressure measurements will then relate differently with age than short-term longitudinal assessments. And it is the latter, measured over real time rather than inferred from single measurements, that is important.

One of the elements complicating the issue of geographical differences in blood pressure is the matter of water hardness, or more precisely, calcium content in drinking water. In general, rural areas have water of low calcium content, and there is a good deal of evidence relating low calcium content to high blood pressures [44]. LANGFORD *et al.* [44] have recently shown that a lower calcium intake in rural Mississippi high school students may be associated with higher pressures. Confirming WALSER's experiments [78]. LANGFORD *et al.* also showed that rats fed low calcium diets and 0.9% saline solution as drinking water developed slightly higher pressures but were both ingesting and excreting almost 50% less sodium than rats fed normal calcium diets. The more calcium available for excretion, the more sodium was excreted. Perhaps, in hard water areas of the world, where calcium intake in drinking water approaches that in food, high calcium intake promotes sodium excretion and tends to lower blood pressures.

Granted that we cannot now answer the question of the meaning of rapid cultural and social change for blood pressures or the rates of rise with age, let us assume for the moment that the relationship are real. Do these studies provide any ideas about the way in which socioeconomic change affects blood pressure. Indeed they do, and the issue has been introduced earlier. Going from a rural traditional way of life to an urban industrial one is fairly predictably associated with an increase in caloric food intake and a fall in caloric expenditure resulting from decreased physical activity. These changes are more characteristic of men undergoing rapid sociocultural change than of women. The changes in food intake and physical activity result in weight gain and the weight gain alone may be sufficient to account for the blood pressure changes.

Our view then is that rapid sociocultural change does, indeed, lead to a higher prevalence of high blood pressure and a greater rise in pressures with age. The intermediary mechanism is a change in diet that causes gain in weight. There is no need to assume that breakdown of traditional social roles and conflict about them directly affect blood pressure.

In a recent elegant review, STUNKARD [79] has examined the relationships between sociocultural variables and obesity. So parallel are these relationships to those between high blood pressure and sociocultural assessments that one can interchange obesity and high blood pressure on charts and tables without losing important information. Obesity in the United States and England is a disease of the poor and uneducated, with no great exceptions [80–82]. It is also a disorder of the immigrants to the United States and their children and its prevalence declines in suceeding generations [83]. In economically deprived societies obesity is a disease of the well educated and affluent. The latter relationship obtained in Latin America, Puerto Rico, South China, the Phillipines and the Navajo of the American Southwest [84–86]. The increased prevalence of obesity is related both to availability of food and to physical activity. In economically deprived societies, the poor and uneducated generally eat fewer calories and expend more at work than the more surfeited and sedentary upper classes [87, 88].

The US Public Health Service population laboratory in Hagerstown, Maryland has provided some data crucially important to our hypothesis [89]. A group of 1,963 white men born between 1910 and 1919 who were studied while in elementary school were contacted for resurvey between 1961 and 1963. Of this total, 1,691 were identified and 717 reexamined. The measurements of concern to us are childhood height and weight, and current blood pressure, height, weight and clinical diagnosis. The highest prevalences of hypertensive vascular disease and cardiovascular renal disease occurred among obese adults who were underweight as children. Those obese in both childhood and adulthood were less afflicted with hypertensive and cardiovascular renal disease as adults.

Persons beginning life in traditional nonindustrial societies who in later life resided in more urbanized industrialized communities have seen great sociocultural change. They are also more likely to have been thin children and overweight adults and thus to be hypertensive and prone to cardiovascular renal disease as adults.

The data reviewed here on obesity and sociocultural variables have the same deficiencies as the blood pressure surveys. They are usually cross-sectional studies and the samples are sometimes inadequate. Here also one may interchange obesity with hypertension and lose little. The sole difference between these surveys is that obesity has been studied comprehensively in children but high blood pressure has not.

The obesity hypothesis is not a very glamorous one. But it is supported by much of the evidence, including most convincingly, the Cape Verdean [66] and Hagerstown [89] studies and buttressed by other data reviewed here. No convincing evidence to refute the hypothesis of weight gain exists, but the hypothesis allows little or no room for considerations of the direct effect on blood pressure of sociocultural stress, or complex central nervous system and endocrine pressor responses to conflict and symbolic threat. The weight gain hypothesis has the enormous advantages of being simple, plausible, consistent with known data, and fairly easily testable. Only long-term longitudinal studies can test it.

Physicians, epidemiologists, and social scientists have demonstrated that only in rare instances are they going to work together on blood pressure problems. And very few social scientists have become interested anyway. So here is an hypothesis internists and epidemiologists can investigate by themselves with the help of biostatisticians. Or biostatisticians can do it with the help of physicians. New opportunities to work with isolated stone age people are still arising in Brazil, the Phillipines and New Guinea.

OSTFELD [90] has written before about the difficulties we all have had in pursuing psychomatic hypotheses in the field of blood pressure. Any bystander who watches the psychosomatic builder can tell him what he is doing wrong. That is not difficult. But that helps only a little. All we can do – all of us – is try again with better methods and sharper hypotheses. High blood pressure remains the most prevalent life threatening disease of man in many parts of the world.

References

1 OSTFELD, A.M. and SHEKELLE, R.B.: Psychosocial variables and blood pressure; in

STAMLER, STAMLER and PULLMAN The epidemiology of hypertension (Grune & Stratton, New York 1967).

2 RUSKIN, A.; BEARD, O.W., and SHAFFER, R.L.: 'Blast hypertension': elevated arterial pressure in victims of the Texas City disaster. Am. J. Med. *4:* 228 (148).

3 GRAHAM, J.D.P.: High blood pressure after battle. Lancet *i:* 239 (1945).

4 LOVELL, R.R.H.; MADDOCKS, I., and ROGERSON, G.W.: The casual arterial pressure of Fijians and Indians in Fiji. Aust. Ann. Med. *9:* 4 (1960).

5 MADDOCKS, I.: The influence of standard of living on blood pressure in Fiji. Abstract. Circulation *24:* 1220 (1961).

6 MADDOCKS, I.: Possible absence of essential hypertension in two complete Pacific Island populations. Lancet *ii:* 396 (1961).

7 KAMINER, B. and LUTZ, W.P.: Blood pressure in Bushmen of the Kalahari desert. Circulation *22:* 289 (1960).

8 POINDEXTER, H.A.: Epidemiologic survey among Gola tribes in Liberia. Am. J. trop. Med. Hyg. *11:* 30 (1953).

9 LOEWENSTEIN, F.W.: Blood pressure in relation to age and sex in the tropics and subtropics. Lancet *i:* 389 (1961).

10 GAMPEL, B.; SLOME, C.; SCOTCH, N., and ABRAMSON, J.: Urbanization and hypertension among Zulu adults. J. chron. Dis. *15:* 67 (1962).

11 SCOTCH, N.A.: Sociocultural factors in the epidemiology of Zulu hypertension. Am. J. publ. Hlth *53:* 1205 (1963).

12 LOVELL, R.R.N.: Blood pressure in Pacific Island populations; in PEMBERTON Epidemiology – reports on research and teaching (Oxford University Press, Fairlawn 1963).

13 KILBORN, L.G.: A note on the blood pressure of primitive races with special reference to the Miao of Kweichow. Chin. J. Physiol. *11:* 135 (1937).

14 MORSE, W.R. and BERG, Y.T.: Blood pressure amongst aboriginal ethnic groups of Szechwan Province, West China, Lancet *i:* 966 (1937).

15 KEAN, B.H.: The blood pressure of the Cuna Indians. Am. J. trop. Med. Hyg. *24:* 341 (1955).

16 LOEWENSTEIN, F.W.: Blood pressure in relation to age and sex in the tropics and subtropics. Lancet *i:* 389 (1961).

17 HICKS, C.S. and MATTERS, R.F.: The standard metabolism of the Australian aborigines. Aust. J. exp. Biol. med. Sci. *11:* 177 (1933).

18 ABBIE, A.A. and SCHROEDER, J.: Blood pressure in Arnhem Land aborigines. Med. J. Aust. *ii:* 493 (1960).

19 POLUNIN, I.: The medical history of Malayan aborigines. Med. J. Malaya *8:* 114 (1953).

20 PADMAVATI, S. and GUPTA, S.: Blood pressure studies in rural and urban groups in Delhi. Circulation *19:* 395 (1959).

21 DONNISON, C.P.: Blood pressure in the African native. Lancet *i:* 6 (1929).

22 ABRAHAMS, D.G.; ALELE, C.A., and BARNARD, B.G.: The systematic blood pressure in a rural West African community. W. Afr. med. J. *9:* 45 (1960).

23 HETZEL, A.M.: Health survey of the Trust Territory of the Pacific Islands. US Armed Forces med. J. *19:* 1199 (1959).

24 HUNTER, J.D.: Diet, body build, Blood pressure and serum cholesterol levels in coconut-eating Polynesians. Fed. Proc. *21:* suppl. 11, p. 36 (1962).

25 PRIOR, I.: A health survey in a rural Maori community with particular emphasis on the cardiovascular, nutritional and metabolic findings. N. Z. med. J. *61:* 333 (1962).

26 WHYTE, H.M.: Body fat and blood pressure of natives in New Guinea. Aust. Ann. Med. *7:* 36 (1958).

27 NORMAN-TAYLOR, W. and REES, W.H.: Blood pressure in three New Hebrides communities. Br. J. prev. soc. Med. *17:* 141 (1963).

28 GOVER, M.: Physical impairments of low-income farm families. publ. Hlth Rep. *63:* 1083 (1948).

29 COMSTOCK, G.W.: An epidemiological study of blood pressure levels in a bi-racial community in the southern United States. Am. J. Hyg. *65:* 271 (1957).

30 MIALL, W.E. and OLDHAM, P.D.: Factors influencing arterial blood pressure in the general population. Clin. Sci. *17:* 409 (1958).

31 DOYLE, A.E. and LOVELL, R.R.H.: Blood pressure and body build in men in tropical and temperate Australia. Clin. Sci. *20:* 243 (1961).

32 SHAPER, A.G.: Blood pressure studies in East Africa; in STAMLER, STAMLER and PULLMAN The epidemiology of hypertension (Grune & Stratton, New York 1967).

33 HENRY, J.P. and CASSEL, J.C.: Psychosocial factors in essential hypertension. Recent epidemiologic and animal experimental studies. Am. J. Epidem. *90:* 171 (1969).

34 FOSTER, J.H.: Practice of medicine in China and New England with observations on hypertension. New Engl. J. Med. *203:* 1073 (1930).

35 OBERMAN, A.; LANE, N.E.; HARLAN, W.R.; GRAYBIEL, A., and MITCHELL, R.E.: Trends in systolic blood pressure in the thousand aviator cohort over a twenty-four year period. Circulation *36:* 812 (1967).

36 HOOBLER, S.W.; TEJADA, C., and PARDO, A.: Influence of nutrition and 'acculturation' on the blood pressure levels and changes with age in the highland Guatemalan Indian. Circulation *31/32:* suppl. 2, p. 1116 (1956).

37 LIN, T.Y.; HUNG, T.; CHEN, C.; HSW, T., and CHEN, K.: A study of normal and elevated blood pressures in a Chinese urban population in Taiwan (Formosa). Clin. Sci. *18:* 301 (1959).

38 SCOTCH, N.A.: An anthropological study of essential hypertension in three societies; Ph.D. thesis, Northwestern University Papers No. 23543 (1957).

39 NISHIMURA, M.; MATSUDA, K.; SUGABARA, J.; WAKISAKA, K.; YOKOTA, M.; HANARTORI, T.; OKUBA, K., and MIKI, K.: On the results of blood pressure measurements of inhabitants in a village in Tottori. Prefect. Jap. Circln. J. *12:* 75 (1948).

40 STROTZ, C.R. and SHORR, G.I.: Hypertension in the Papago Indien. Circulation *48:* 1299 (1973).

41 TENBRINCK, M.S.: Blood pressure comparisons in tropical Africans and Peruvians. III. White Mountain Apaches of Arizona compared with Shepibos of Peru. N.Y. St. J. Med. *1968:* 1132.

42 TSENG, W.: Blood pressure and hypertension in an agricultural and a fishing population in Taiwan. Am. J. Epidem. *86:* 513 (1967).

43 D'ATRI, D. and OSTFELD, A.: Crowding: its effects on the elevation of blood pressure in a prison setting. Prev. Med. *4:* 550–556 (1975).

44 LANGFORD, H.G.; WATSON, R.L., and DOUGLAS, B.: Factors affecting blood pressure in population groups. Trans. Ass. Am. Physns *5:* 135 (1970).

45 MIALL, W.E. and COCHRANE, A.L.: The distribution of arterial pressure in Wales and Jamaica. Pathol. Microbiol. *24:* 690 (1961).

46 REID, D.D.; HOLLAND, W.W.; HUMERFELT, S., and ROSE, G.A.: Cardiovascular survey of British postal workers. Lancet *i:* 614 (1966).

47 Vital and Health Statistics: Data from the National Health Survey Blood Pressure of Adults by Race and Area. PHS Pub. 1000, Series II, No. 5.

48 McDONOUGH, J.R.: Blood pressure and hypertensive diseases among Negroes and whites. Ann. intern. Med. *61:* 208 (1964).

49 KULLER, L.: Nationwide cerebrovascular disease mortality study. Stroke *1:* 86 (1970).

50 HEYMAN, A., *et al.:* Cerebrovascular disease in the biracial population of Evans County, Georgia. Stroke *26:* 509 (1971).

51 National Center for Health Statistics: Blood pressures of adults by race and area. Vital and Health Statistics, PHS Pub. No. 1000, Series II, No. 4 (US Government Printing Office, Washington 1966).

52 WILBER, G.L. and ROGERS, T.W.: Interstate migration of the Mississipi population 1960. Mississippi State University Agricultural Experiment Station Bull. No. 717 (1965).

53 BRYANT, E.S. and WILBER, G.L.: Net migration in Mississippi 1950 to 1960. Mississippi State University Agricultural Experiment Station Bull. No. 632 (1961).

54 BRYANT, E.S.: Mississippi county population estimates by race and age 1965. Mississippi State University Agricultural Experiment Station Sociology and Rural Life Series No. 17 (1966).

55 SHIMKIN, D.B.: Black migration and the struggle for equity. A hundred year equity; in EATON Migration and social welfare. New York Nat. Ass. Soc. Wk. Inc. (1971).

56 OSTFELD, A.M. and SHIMKIN, D.B.: Planning Conference on the Ecology of Migrant Populations of the Sectional Committee on the International Biological Program, Chicago, Ill. (National Academy of Sciences, Washington 1967).

57 LEE, E.S.: A theory of migration. Demography *3:* 47 (1966).

58 JORGENSON, R.J.; BOLLING, D.R.; YODER, O.C., and MURPHY, E.A.: Blood pressure studies in the Amish. Hopkins med. J. *131:* 329 (1972).

59 JOHNSON, T.O.: Arterial pressures and hypertension in an urban African population sample. Br. J. prev. soc. Med. *25:* 26 (1971).

60 MASTER, A.M.; DUBLIN, L.I., and MARKS, H.H.: The normal blood pressure range and its clinical applications. J. Am. med. Ass. *143:* 1464 (1950).

61 BØE, J.; HUMERFELT, S., and WEDERVANG, F.: The Blood pressure in a population. Acta med. scand., suppl. 321 (1957).

62 HAMILTON, H.; PICKERING, G.W.; ROBERTS, J.A.F., and SOWRY, G.S.: Arterial pressures of relatives of patients with secondary and Malignant hypertension. Clin. Sci. *24:* 91 (1963).

63 JOHNSON, B.C.; EPSTEIN, F.H., and KJELSBERG, M.O.: Distributions and familial studies of blood pressure and serum cholesterol levels in a total community – Tecumseh, Michigan. J. chron. Dis. *18:* 147 (1965).

64 PRIOR, I.; STANHOPE, J.; EVANS, J., and SALMOND, C.: The Tokelau Island migrant study. Int. J. Epidem. *3:* 225 (1974).

65 PRIOR, I.: Cardiovascular epidemiology in New Zealand and the Pacific. N. Z. med. J. *80:* 245 (1974).

66 Florey, C. du V. and Cuadrado, R.R.: Blood pressure in native Cape Verdeans and in Cape Verdean immigrants and their descendants living in New England. Hum. Biol. *40:* 189 (1968).

67 Kannel, W.B. Brand, N.; Skinner, J.J.; Dawber, T.R., and McNamara, P.M.: The relationship of adiposity to blood pressure and development of hypertension. The Framingham study. Ann. intern. Med. *67:* 48 (1967).

68 Whyte, H.M.: Blood pressure and obesity. Circulation *19:* 511 (1959).

69 Pickering, G.W.: High blood pressure (Churchill, London 1955).

70 Smirk, F.H.: High arterial pressure (Blackwell, Oxford 1957).

71 Robinson, S.C.; Brucer, M., and Mass, J.: Hypertension and obesity. J. Lab. clin. Med. *25:* 807 (1940).

72 Thomas, C.B. and Cohen, B.H.: The familial occurrence of hypertension and coronary artery disease with observations concerning obesity and diabetes. Ann. intern. Med. *42:* 90 (1955).

73 Bjerkedal, T.: Overweight and hypertension. Acta med. scand. *159:* 13 (1951).

74 Levy, R.L.; White, P.D.; Stroud, W.D., and Hamilton, C.C.: Overweight: its prognostic significance in relation to hypertension and cardiovascular renal diseases. J. Am. med. Ass. *131:* 951 (1946).

75 Fletcher, A.P.: The effect of weight reduction upon the blood pressure of obese hypertensive women. Q. Jl Med. *23:* 331 (1959).

76 Kagan, A.; Gordon, T.; Kannel, W.B., and Dawber, T.R.: Blood pressure and its relationship to coronary heart disease in Framingham study. Proc. Coun. high Blood Press. Res. *7:* 53 (1959).

77 Paul, O.; Lepper, M.; Phelan, W.; Dupertius, G.; MacMillan, A.; McKean, H., and Park, H.: A longitudinal study of coronary heart disease. Circulation *28:* 20 (1963).

78 Walser, M.: Ion association. VII. Dependence of calciuresis on natriuresis during sulfate infusion. Am. J. Physiol. *201:* 769 (1961).

79 Stunkard, A.J.: From explanation to action in psychosomatic medicine. The case of obesity. Psychosom. Med. *37:* 195 (1975).

80 Hueneman, R.L.: Factors association with teenage obesity; in Wilson Obesity (Davies, Philadelphia 1969).

81 Whitelaw, G.L.: Association of social class and sibling number with skinfold thickness in London school boys. Hum. Biol. *43:* 414 (1971).

82 Stunkard, A.J.; d'Asquili, E., and Fox, S., *et al.:* The influence of social class on obesity and thinness in children. J. Am. med. Ass. *221:* 579 (1972).

83 Goldblatt, P.B.; Moore, M.E., and Stunkard, A.J.: Social factors in obesity. J. Am. med. Ass. *192:* 1039 (1965).

84 Baily, K.: The study of human growth in the framework of applied nutrition and public health nutrition programs in the western Pacific region in physical growth and body composition; in Brozek Kyato Symposium on Anthropological Aspects of Human Growth. Monogr. Soc. Res. Child. Dev. vol. 35, p. 7 (University of Chicago Press, Chicago 1970).

85 Chang, K.S.; Lee, M.M.; Law, W.D., *et al.:* Height and weight of southern Chinese children in Hong Kong. Am. J. phys. Anthrop. *21:* 497 (1963).

86 Garh, J.L.; Garh, J.R., and Stunkard, A.J.: The influence of social factors on

obesity and thinness in Navajo children. Abst. 1st Int. Congr. on Obesity, Royal College of Physicians, London 1974.

87 WEST, K.M.: Epidemiology of adiposity in regulation of adipose tissue mass. Proc. 4th Int. Conf. Meet. of Endocrinology 1973, pp. 202–207 (Excerpta Medica, Amsterdam 1974).

88 MAYER, J.: The role of exercise and activity in weight control; in EPPRIGHT, SWANSON and IVERSON Weight control (Iowa State College Press, Ames 1955).

89 ABRAHAM, S.; COLLINS, G., and NORDSIECK, M.: Relationship of childhood weight status to morbidity in adults. HSMHA Hlth Rep. *86:* 273–284 (1971).

90 OSTFELD, A.M.: What's the payoff in hypertension research. Psychosom. Med. *35:* No. 1 (1973).

Dr. A.M. OSTFELD, Department of Epidemiology and Public Health, Yale University School of Medicine, *New Haven, CT 06513* (USA)

Adv. psychosom. Med., vol. 9, pp. 38–47 (Karger, Basel 1977)

The Prevalence of Anorexia nervosa and Some of Its Associations in the General Population

A.H. Crisp

Department of Psychiatry, University of London, at St. George's Hospital Medical School, Tooting, London

Contents

Until recently anorexia nervosa has been regarded as a rare disorder. Investigators have now begun to publish reports of large series of patients [1–7] and there is a view that the condition may be getting more common [1–3, 6, 9–11]. In the past there has been disagreement over the necessary diagnostic criteria for and the nature of the disorder. This is now largely resolved, but since many subjects deny the true nature of their illness both to themselves and to others and conceal from others much of the behaviour rooted in it, clinical studies and especially would-be survey studies can still expect to be fraught with the problems of recognition and differentiation of the state. As a consequence also the differential diagnosis is particularly complex and many patients languish in medical and psychiatric care misclassified, for instance as cases of unexplained functional vomiting, diarrhoea, abdominal pain or amenorrhea, periodic fluid retention, obscure endocrine syndromes or atypical psychiatric syndromes of one or other variety.

Against this background it is perhaps surprising that certain clinical features stand out seemingly beyond dispute. There is universal agreement that the disorder presents itself much more frequently in females than males. The sex ratio is probably of the order of 20 to 1 [12]. Furthermore, it is clear that by far the commonest age of onset, whether this be taken in retro-

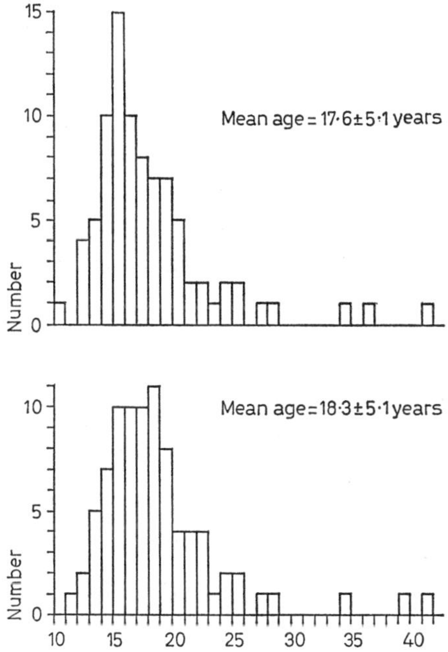

Fig. 1. Age at onset of severe dieting behaviour (a) and LMP (b) in 86 patients with anorexia nervosa. Reproduced by kind permission, Editor, *British Medical Journal* [14].

spect to have been the point at which the pathological dietary carbohydrate restriction first occurred or else the age at which amenorrhea supervened, is in adolescence (fig. 1).

Most clinicians also find that their patients frequently come from a high socio-economic class background, more so than is the case with their other patients. It is unlikely that this is due to clinic or personal selection factors. Premorbid obesity is a common feature [2, 6, 8, 13, 14], as is a history of disorders of weight, which include anorexia nervosa and psychiatric illness of a neurotic avoidance and depressive kind, in the families and particularly the parents [2, 12, 15–17]. Moreover, obese subjects and subjects with psychiatric illness in the third, fourth and later decades of life sometimes give a history of a period of undiagnosed anorexia nervosa during their adolescence if careful enquiries are made [18], being more able by this stage to recognise this condition in themselves and to reveal the facts to others.

Other Clinical Features

The disorder is almost invariably rooted in an initial wish to lose weight which leads to early attempts to eliminate carbohydrate from the diet. In the subject who develops anorexia nervosa this behaviour has become excessive – the gonadotrophic endocrine processes activated by puberty have ceased, this being declared clinically by amenorrhea and atrophy of secondary sex genital characteristics, and in laboratory terms by the absence of gonadotrophins in the urine [5] and in the blood [19]. Physical growth will decelerate or cease if the disorder has arisen before its completion. The features of starvation will be present – emaciation, absence of subcutaneous fat, reduced cardiac output, hypothermia and hirsutism, all usually characterised metabolically by the carbohydrate starvation and its effects. The resistance to eating in the face of continued hunger may continue for some while and is usually denied. The emaciated subject develops an intense fear of even limited weight gain, refuses under any circumstances to contemplate weight gain above about 45 kg, and begins to increasingly overestimate her present size when asked about the latter. It has been suggested that the disorder reflects a psychosomatic avoidance response to the maturational demands and conflicts generated in the family and the subject by the latter's adolescence. The resolution of this conflict throught the subject's biological regression which probably occurs around a critical weight threshold [20], continually reinforces and intensifies the dieting behaviour.

The natural history of the condition is one which ranges from natural recovery through to chronicity, sometimes including secondary more complicated feeding patterns of indiscriminate eating followed by vomiting and purging. When death occurs it is usually through inanition or suicide. An episode of illness can last for just a few months but usually the disorder lasts for several years. Physical recovery can occur but so can relapse in middle life if the pre-occupations with weight and shape are unabated or rekindled.

Since the disorder is rooted in dieting behaviour it is perhaps not surprising that premorbid obesity is over-represented in the population of patients (fig. 2).

Furthermore, this often reflects a long-standing state associated with high birth weight and being later born [13]. Such premorbid obesity may of course itself have certain experiential determinants of a 'neurotic' kind and, in the population at large, is also likely to have been associated with a high growth rate, early puberty [21] and hence more rapid than usual

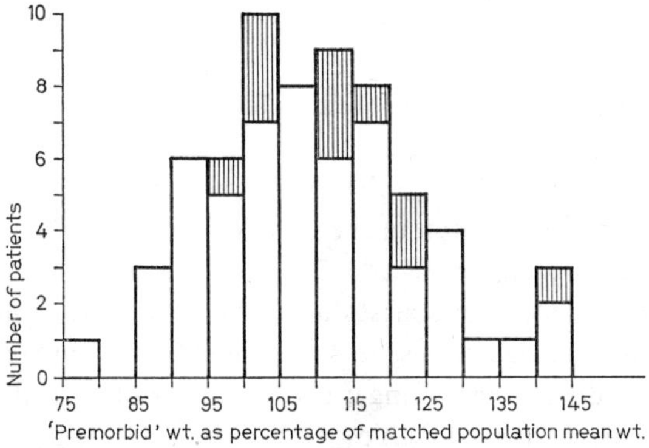

Fig. 2. 'Premorbid' (i.e. onset of dieting) weight as percentage of matched population mean weight in 65 patients with anorexia nervosa. □ = 54 patients on whom full clinical data are available. Reproduced by kind permission, Editor, *British Medical Journal* [14].

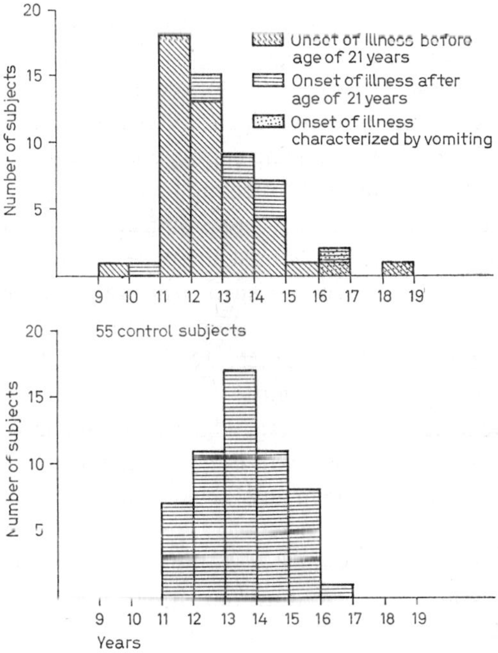

Fig. 3. Distribution of reported recollected menarchal ages of anorexia nervosa and control subjects. Reproduced by kind permission, Editor, *Journal of Psychosomatic Research* [13].

precipitation into adolescence. This phenomenon is shown clearly within the anorexia nervosa clinic population [3] whose premorbid obesity as a group is associated with significantly early menarche when compared with the matched non-anorectic population (fig. 3).

High growth rate and related greater plumpness in the general population and puberty are also more common in the female than the male and in both sexes are getting earlier decade by decade [22]. Meanwhile, FRISCH *et al.* [23] have clearly shown that menarche arises at a critical weight of about 47 kg irrespective of height or age. Thus, to take the extremes, puberty is likely to overtake an individual either younger and plump or older and thin. Once into adolescence, the nature of adolescent experience is again substantially different between the sexes. In this situation the female's shape is the focus of attention especially if it changes. Thus we have a number of features of a biological and experiential kind which differentiate the female from the male at adolescence and which come together to contribute to sex differences concerning attitudes to weight and shape.

There ar now also some relevant general population studies of adolescent attitudes to weight and shape and of related behaviour. Thus HUENEMANN *et al.* [24] studied approximately 1,000 teenagers in the USA Public High School system over a 4-year period. These investigators combined an anthropometric study with careful questionnaire investigation regarding teenagers' preferences, views and knowledge about food and eating, body conformation and activity. Fewer girls than boys admitted to feeling hungry; they ate less and about 50% classified themselves as obese whereas only 25% were identified as obese in anthropometric terms. In contrast the male population did not overestimate its fatness in comparison to such measures. The males' main concern at all ages was to gain weight and/or size and also to gain strength. To the extent that they sought to control weight they preferred to achieve this through exercise. In contrast the girls' main priority was to lose weight and to attempt to achieve this by dieting. This was particularly true of obese girls. These findings are in accord with everyday experience. Thus dieting behaviour is endemic and epidemic in girls' schools and rarely occurs in boys' schools.

Another epidemiological study, this time of Scandinavian school girls [25] brings us closer to the issure of anorexia nervosa itself.

NYLANDER [25] studied a group of 2,370 subjects aged 14–19 years (1,129 boys and 1,241 girls) in the Swedish town of Umea during the year 1970. They comprised children in the primary schools, the local college for higher education and the local technical or trades school. The design of the study had the effect of including nearly all 16 year olds in the town, one quarter of the town's 14 and 15 year olds and all the pupils attending the two senior schools (i.e. the majority of 18–19 year olds and somewhat fewer 20 and 21 year olds). NYLANDER was satisfied that his sample was truly representative. Investigation was conducted primarily by questionnaires administered under supervision. Weight and height data were obtained by this route and in addition through the school health records of every fourth subject.

Most of the girls in this study reported that at some time they had felt fat (although obesity in terms of overweight was not a marked feature of the overall population). This feeling as a current phenomenon was most common among the 18 year olds (50%) but was already present in 26% of the 14 year olds. A minority of males (e.g. 7% at the age of 18 years) reported similar feelings and, unlike the females, the proportion grew slightly but steadily greater with age (e.g., 9% at 20 years, 16% at 21 years of age), at which point, however, the sample was probably not truly representative of the general population.

Of the girls who thought that they were fat many had attempted to diet (e.g., 10% of 14 year olds, 40% of 18 year olds). Boys seldom reported dieting. The frequency amongst the girls was twice as high amongst those whose weight was above the mean for their representative heights. Thus 76% of 18 year olds in this latter category were on a diet. The majority of them also reported dieting because they felt fat although some wrote that it was because they had felt ill and attributed this to their fatness. In the majority of cases it was reported that dieting had openly resulted in minor weight loss but the number of subjects reporting a loss of more than 5 kg increased with age. Overall, 151 subjects reported such a loss as having occurred at some stage.

A total of 119 cases (12 boys, 107 girls) reported that they had developed at least three of the following symptoms in connection with the loss of weight: anxiety, depression, anxiety associated with meals, increased interest in food and food preparation, chilliness, constipation, amenorrhea (at least three months' interruption), that they had become mentally sluggish and slow performed less well in school, or had less zest and interest in things that had previously interested them. Overall, 34 girls reported amenorrhea whilst dieting. Meanwhile, 15 of the 107 girls who reported three or more of the above symptoms also reported that they had lost 10 kg or more in weight; of these 10 reported that they had dieted repeatedly and for long periods. Eight of the 107 were known to the child psychiatric clinic as cases of anorexia nervosa.

Approximately 1 in 10 of both males and females in this study also reported having lost weight at some stage without dieting and this had arisen about equally in all age groups. Finally, some subjects reported feeling too thin but this was particularly uncommon in the female 17- to 18-year-old range. NYLANDER concludes by stating that, if mild cases are included, it can be said that approximately 1 in 10 of the girls in his study reported experiencing an anorexia nervosa like syndrome. Certainly it would appear that as many as 1 in 150 quite unequivocally had the disorder, it being independently diagnosed in the clinic. NYLANDER has the view that the syndrome may not have profound psychopathological determinants. He identifies the feeling of being fat as a predeterminant but does not feel obliged to explore the meaning of this further or to consider whether the intensive and sustained dieting which develops to underpin the evolution of the syndrome implied some further meaningful over-determination and reinforcement of such behaviour.

Meanwhile, in a related study conducted together with a gynaecological colleague [26], the authors concluded once again that the syndrome is very much more common than is supposed. They found that of 54 consecutive women presenting with secondary amenorrhea, after intensive investigations, the most significant finding in 51 subjects was a concurrent loss of weight (11 kg average, range 3–28 kg) at about the time of the last menstrual period. Furthermore, 41 of these subjects had symptoms characteristic of anorexia nervosa.

Another study by RUSSELL [27] also serves to demonstrate that the condition, especially in its milder forms is probably common. RUSSELL started by comparing a group of female anorexia nervosa patients with a population of females of comparable age drawn from local schools (day and boarding) and a college. He found that the patients were significantly more often (1) of social class I and II family background, (2) boarding school educated, (3) later born in family, (4) geographically mobile, (5) bereaved of the maternal grandmother before the age of 10 years. Amongst the 'normal' subjects, 15% reported weight loss of 7 lb. or more, 6% reported amenorrhea of at least 6 months' duration and 4% reported both these. Furthermore, this latter group was found to contain a significantly high proportion who reported experiencing three or more of the above social factors which he had identified as characterising the clinic patients with anorexia nervosa.

Such a figure of 4% is substantially in excess even of the high prevalence of the disorder of between 1 and 2% in females of this age range and social class background, as suggested by CRISP and TOMS [12]. The same authors also suggested a male prevalence rate of about 0.1% .However, they were concerned with apparent and severe cases and obtained their data by asking each patient with the condition how many other individuals with the same disorder she was aware of in her school. DUDDLE [11], working in a university health centre, is also impressed with the high incidence, having 13 new cases referred to her in 1971. There is a strong impression amongst many clinicians that the condition is getting more common especially in the clinic setting [11, 28] and there are plausible explanations for this, e.g., increasing over-nutrition in our society, increasingly early puberty especially amongst females, and also the increasing need for self-imposed controls of behaviour in adolescence as social controls lessen. However, it is important to remember that school teachers with experience of adolescent school girls, going back over several decades, will often say that the condition has always been fairly common.

Summary

Anorexia nervosa is a common condition amongst adolescent females especially those from higher socio-economic backgrounds. The prevalence is at present probably about one in every hundred of this population. It is much more rare amongst adolescent males, in whom the rate is likely to be one in every two thousand or so individuals. Immediate premorbid factors of the clinic population of anorexia nervosa patients include actual obesity and almost invariably include dieting behaviour. Adolescent obesity is common, is getting commoner and is associated with high growth rate and early puberty and precipitation into adolescence especially amongst females. Subsequent dieting is commonplace amongst the adolescent female population and this is in contrast to the behaviour of adolescent males. The psychosocial maturational demands of adolescence also remain importantly different between the sexes. This triad of immediate factors probably contributes substantially to the major difference in prevalence of the condition between the sexes and may also account for its apparent increase.

References

1 THOMA, H.: Anorexia nervosa (International Universities Press, New York 1967).
2 DALLY, P.: Anorexia nervosa (Heinemann, London 1969).
3 CRISP, A.H.: Anorexia nervosa 'feeding disorder', 'nervous malnutrition' or 'weight phobia'? Wld Rev. Nutr. Diet. *12:* 452–504 (1970).
4 ROWLAND, C.V.: Anorexia and obesity. International psychiatry clinics, vol. 7, No. 1 (Little, Brown, Boston 1970).
5 RUSSELL, G.F.M.: Anorexia nervosa: its identity as an illness and its treatment; in

Price Modern trends in psychological medicine, chap. 6 (Butterworth, London 1970).

6 Theander, S.: Anorexia nervosa. Acta psychiat. scand., supp. 214 (1970).

7 Meyer, J.E.: Anorexia nervosa of adolescence. The central syndrome of the anorexia nervosa group. Br. J. Psychiat. *118:* 539–542 (1971).

8 Bruch, H.: Eating disorders (Routledge & Kegan, London 1974).

9 Bruch, H.: Anorexia nervosa and its differential diagnosis. J. nerv. ment. Dis. *141:* 555–566 (1965).

10 Sours, J.A.: Anorexia nervosa: nosology, diagnosis, developmental patterns and power-control dynamics; in Caplan and Lebovici Adolescence: psychosocial perspectives, pp. 185–212 (Basic Books, New York 1969).

11 Duddle, M.: An increase of anorexia nervosa in a university population. Br. J. Psychiat. *123:* 711–712 (1973).

12 Crisp, A.H. and Toms, D.A.: Primary anorexia nervosa or weight phobia in the male. Report on 13 cases. Br. med. J. *i:* 334–338 (1972).

13 Crisp, A.H.: Reported birth weights and growth rates in a group of patients with primary anorexia nervosa (weight phobia). J. psychosom. Res. *14:* 23–50 (1970).

14 Crisp, A.H. and Stonehill, E.: Relation between aspects of nutritional disturbance and menstrual activity in primary anorexia nervosa. Br. med. J. *i:* 149–151 (1971).

15 Crisp, A.H.: Some aspects of the evolution, presentation and follow-up of anorexia nervosa. Proc. R. Soc. Med. *58:* 814–820 (1965).

16 Crisp, A.H.: Anorexia nervosa. Hosp. med. *1967:* 713–718.

17 Kay, D.W.K. and Leigh, D.: The natural history, treatment and prognosis of anorexia nervosa, based on a study of 38 patients. J. ment. Sci. *100:* 411–431 (1954).

18 Crisp, A.H.: The possible significance of some behavioural correlates of weight and carbohydrate intake. J. psychosom. Res. *11:* 117–131 (1967).

19 Crisp, A.H.; Chen, C.; Mackinnon, P.C.B., and Corker, C.S.: Observations of gonadotrophic and ovarian hormone activity during recovery from anorexia nervosa. Postgrad. med. J. *49:* 584–590 (1973).

20 Crisp, A.H.: The nature of primary anorexia nervosa. R. Coll. Physician, Edin., Pubn. No. 42, pp 18–30 (1971).

21 Crisp, A.H.; Douglas, J.W.R.; Ross, J.M., and Stonehill, E.: Some developmental aspects of disorders of weight. J. psychosom. Res. *14:* 313–320 (1970).

22 Tanner, J.M.: Growth at adolescence; 2nd ed. (Blackwell, Oxford 1962).

23 Frisch, R.E.; Revelle, R., and Cook, S.: Height, weight and age at menarche and the 'critical weight' hypothesis. Science *174:* 1148–1149 (1972).

24 Huenemann, R.L.; Shapiro, L.R.; Hampton, M.C., and Mitchell, B.W.: A longitudinal study of gross body composition and body conformation and their association with food and activity in a teenage population. Am. J. clin. Nutr. *18:* 325–338 (1966).

25 Nylander, I.: The feeling of being fat and dieting in a school population. Epidemiologic interview investigation. Acta sociomed. scand. *3:* 17–26 (1971).

26 Holmberg, N.G. and Nylander, I.: Weight loss in secondary amenorrhea. Acta obstet. gynec. scand. *50:* 241–246 (1971).

27 RUSSELL, J.A.O.: Psychosocial aspects of weight loss and amenorrhea in adolescent girls; in MORRIS Psychosomatic medicine in obstetrics and Gynaecology, pp. 593–595 (Karger, Basel 1971).
28 KENDELL, R.E.; HALL, D.J.; HAILEY, A., and BABIGIAN, H.M.: The epidemiology of anorexia nervosa. Psychol. Med. *3:* 200–203 (1973).

A.H. CRISP, Professor of Psychiatry, University of London, at St. George's Hospital Medical School, Tooting, *London SW 17* (England)

Adv. psychosom. Med., vol. 9, pp. 48–62 (Karger, Basel 1977)

Epidemiologic Aspects of Anorexia nervosa

OSCAR W. HILL

Department of Psychiatry, Middlesex Hospital, London

Contents

The clinical aspects of anorexia nervosa have been described at length in an earlier volume of this series by SEAVER and BINDER [1972], KAY and SCHAPIRA [1972] and THOMA [1972]. The epidemiology of anorexia nervosa has only recently become the object of enquiry. It has for long been regarded as a curiosity and rarity. It is only in the last 20 years that it has been seen and recognised with such frequency that it has become a proper subject for major investigation. An essential feature of epidemiological investigation is the ascertainment of the factors that promote disease in the community at large. It can also legitimately and usefully identify the factors that determine why a segment only of the sick population comes forward for medical help. What we must try to avoid is to muddle these two sets of determinants. The way in which a sick person becomes a patient has clearly been described in an earlier volume of this series [LIPOWSKI, 1972].

The distinction is particularly important in anorexia nervosa as there is probably no disease with such serious physical consequences in which the sick person is so reluctant to come for help and is so unwilling to even recognise that there is a problem. Characteristically these patients usually come to clinicians because of the insistence of parents or from gynaecologists to whom they have gone because of their amenorrhoea. In THEANDER's [1970] series, of the 9 patients who died, 6 died at home or very soon after admission to hospital, reflecting how these patients may fiercely hold out against any acceptance of medical help even in the face of impending death.

Criteria for Diagnosis

A fundamental requirement for epidemiological studies is agreement on the criteria for diagnosis. However, there is a wide divergence of opinion on the criteria for the diagnosis of anorexia nervosa. FEIGHNER *et al.* [1972] have drawn up guidelines which seem to have gained some acceptance in the USA.

These criteria are[1]:

Onset before 25 years of age
Anorexia with accompanying weight loss of at least 25% of original body weight
A distorted, implacable attitude toward eating, food, or weight that overrides hunger, admonitions, reassurance, and threats, for example:
    Denial of illness, with a failure to recognise nutritional needs
    Apparent enjoyment in losing weight, with the overt manifestation that food refusal is pleasurable indulgence
A desired body image of extreme thinness, with overt evidence that it is rewarding to the patient to achieve and maintain this state
Unusual hoarding or handling of food
No known medical illness that could account for the anorexia and weight loss
No other known psychiatric disorder, with particular reference to primary affective disorders, schizophrenia, obsessive-compulsive and phobic neurosis is assumed that, even though it may appear phobic or obsessional, food refusal alone is not sufficient to qualify for obsessive-compulsive or phobic disease)
At least two of the following manifestations:
    Amenorrhoea
    Lanugo
    Bradycardia (persistent resting pulse of 60 or less)

1 The author wants to point out that some of the following criteria are more important than others and, furthermore, that this list does not take into account that certain symptoms need to occur rather closely in time with each other, before they can be counted as criteria.

Periods of overactivity
Episodes of bulimia
Vomiting (may be self-induced)

It must be borne in mind that these criteria could be satisfied only by a fairly severe case of anorexia nervosa and their strict application is likely to err on the side of making sure that no doubtful cases are included, but almost certainly would mean the omission of many patients who would clinically be judged to have anorexia nervosa. For example a patient whose illness is developing will not be accepted as having anorexia nervosa in this scheme until she has reached the later stages of the illness. Probably the only way round this difficulty is to recognise the arbitrary nature of any cut-off point but to hope that all workers will clearly define their criteria. An alternative view is that of SELVINI [1965] and BRUCH [1965, 1966] who give a central place to the clinical evaluation in deciding whether a patient has anorexia nervosa, 'a highly clinical operation' as SELVINI has described it, putting the emphasis on the patient's attitudes rather than on her behaviour. BRUCH has typified anorexia nervosa as 'a struggle for control, for a sense of identity and effectiveness, with relentless pursuit of thinness as a final step in this effort', The central importance of thinness as against the avoidance of eating has been asserted by CRISP who has proposed that the illness be renamed 'weight phobia'.

Incidence

THEANDER [1970] identified 90 female patients who had been admitted to hospital over a 30-year period, giving a crude yearly incidence of 3.1 cases. The population served is 1.3 million giving an incidence of 0.24/100,000 inhabitants. As THEANDER points out, his material shows a rising incidence over the years and the incidence calculated from his last decade (1951–1960) gives 0.45 cases per 100,000. His study is devoted to hospitalised patients and it seems likely that during the 30 years a substantial number of patients were seen in clinics and because they were not later hospitalised were lost to the series. To the extent that even his group of 'mild cases' lost an average of 25% of their pre-morbid body weight, he was dealing with the more severely ill end of the spectrum.

All clinical studies suffer the very serious disadvantage that they include only patients who have been referred for help and some are even more restricted to those who have been referred for help to a psychiatrist. In THEANDER's [1970] study, over a third of the patients were never seen by a psychiatrist. Recently, KENDELL *et al.* [1973] have ascertained and compared the incidence of anorexia nervosa in three psychiatric case registers kept in North-East Scotland (1963–1971), Monroe County USA (1960–1969) and Camberwell, England (1965–1971). In the Scottish region, with a population of $^1/_2$ million there were 47 cases (44 female, 3 male), giving a crude incidence of 1.6/100,000 per year or taking just the female population aged 15–34 an incidence of 10/100,000 per year. In Monroe County the population studied was $^2/_3$ million, nearly all white. There were 24 cases (17 female, 7 male) making a crude incidence of 0.37/100,000 per year or taking just the female population aged 15–34, 0.8/100,000. This unusually low figure is due to the atypical skewing of the age of their patients in that 8 were less than 15 years old and 3 were over 34 when their illnesses were identified and recorded on the register (all female), making an incidence of 0.66/100,000 inhabitants and 4.1/100,000 females aged 15–34. In Camberwell, no cases at all were recorded in the first half of the survey period, for which the explanation can only be conjectural. Unfortunately, factors such as the extent to which the physicians in a region manage anorexia nervosa patients without habitually asking for psychiatric help and the change in such attitudes may have a mojar distorting effect on this type of enquiry. The extent to which younger patients are represented is also capricious especially where the provision of in-patient child psychiatric facilities are meagre. A similar bias is reflected in clinical studies, for example, HALMI [1974] has found 39% of her patients to be 15 or under at the onset of their illness a figure comparable with the Monroe County finding but she attributes this weighting to her having searched the paediatric files for cases.

MORGAN and SYLVESTER [1974] studied 728 18-year-old female students who came to the University of Bristol in October 1973. They initially obtained a routine medical questionnaire from each patient, countersigned by the student's family doctor and then personally interviewed all students who on the basis of the questionnaire, may have at some time suffered an episode of anorexia nervosa. They ascertained that at some time in their lives (some currently), 15 of the students had developed anorexia nervosa. This gives a rate of 2%. The rate is much higher than has been suggested in the clinical studies. As well as being inflated by the inclusion of cases that had not made contact with hospital services, it is likely that these students come more from social classes I, II and III in which anorexia nervosa appears to be more prevalent.

On the other hand, at the age of 18 these individuals have not completed the period of risk for anorexia nervosa so that the final lifetime risk is likely to be greater.

RUSSELL [1972] received completed questionnaires from 110 school girls (aged 16–18) and 121 nurses and female medical students. Among the items for which he made enquiry were a weight loss of 7 lb. or more and secondary amenorrhoea loss and 6% had amenorrhoea as defined. 4% of the respondents had experienced a combination of the two items. He has other data which strengthens the view that this 4% may be seen as suffering an episode, albeit mildly, of anorexia nervosa.

Anorexia nervosa in Males

The difficulties of epidemiological work in the field of anorexia nervosa are highlighted when we consider the male. Certain diagnostic criteria employed by some workers, amenorrhoea obviously, cannot be used in male patients, of course.

Others such as SELVINI [1965] do not deny the possibility but assert that they have not seen a true case of the illness in a male but that the gross loss of weight with disturbance of eating has always been secondary to other forms of psychiatric disorder.

In recent years the conviction has grown that there is in males, a syndrome of anorexia nervosa indistinguishable in all features (apart of course from amenorrhoea) from that found in females.

BEUMONT *et al.* [1972] reviewed the literature on male anorexia nervosa. Of the 250 cases of psychogenic inanition they found, 25 satisfied rigorous contemporary criteria for the diagnosis. Many others were clearly not anorexia nervosa, but there was also a considerable number in which the data presented were insufficient to come to a firm conclusion. They also described 6 cases of their own. BRUCH [1971] has reported 9 male patients (5 with primary anorexia nervosa and 4 atypical ones) not included in the above review. CRISP and TOMS [1972] have published descriptions of 13 cases. Most psychiatrists with an interest in anorexia nervosa have seen a number of male cases – the present author has had 3 under his care. There are some apparent differences in the natural history of the illness in the two sexes. The onset appears rather earlier in the male. Combining the 48 cases for which age of onset is available in the publications by BEUMONT *et al.* [1972], BRUCH [1971] and CRISP and TOMS [1972], 30 patients, i.e. 60% became ill first between the ages of 11 and 15 with a peak at 12. THEANDER's [1970] female patients had a peak age of onset aged 17–18 and HALMI's [1974] peak was between 16 and 25. Most authors are agreed that the prognosis is worse in the male.

Relative Frequency of Anorexia nervosa in the Two Sexes

CRISP and TOMS [1972] had 11 males referred to them during which period of time 160 females were referred to the same service, i.e. a ratio of 1:15. The studies of KENDELL *et al.* [1973] revealed a ratio of 1:15 in NE Scotland, of 2:5 in Monroe County, while no male cases were recorded in Camberwell as against 8 females. ROWLAND [1970] in his series had 6 males and 24 females a ratio of 1:4. The incidence of male anorexia nervosa is very likely to be underreported as it lacks the very obvious symptom of amenorrhoea that so often gives the impetus for seeking help in female subjects. Thus, the vagaries and special circumstances that operate in anorexia nervosa bringing the person into contact with medical agencies are likely to result in an even greater variability of male than female statistics.

Is the Incidence of Anorexia nervosa Increasing?

There is a general agreement that doctors are seeing more cases now but considerable uncertainty whether this reflects a true increase in the incidence of the disease or an increasing likelihood of recognition and referral of an affected person.

In THEANDER's [1970] material the numbers referred in successive decades between 1931 to 1960 were 11, 25 and 58.

In the case register study of KENDELL *et al.* [1973] each of the three centres had more patients registered in the second half of the observation period, the actual figures being in Scotland a ratio of 10:20, in Monroe County of 9:15 and in Camberwell of 0:08. THEANDER made a comparison between the groups of patients admitted in each decade and found no statistically significant difference between them except that the earlier patients were more severely ill. It can only remain speculative whether this change is a reflection of increasing recognition of the disease by physicians and of referral habits than of an increasing incidence of the disease.

Although it does not achieve statistical significance, there is a well-defined trend for more recent patients to come from a lower social class.

The interpretation of this trend is open to speculation. It may be due to the greater availability and acceptability of medical services to the disadvantaged so that cases which would have otherwise remained unidentified in the community come forward for medical help. Alternatively, with the general increase of affluence in the west, the way of life of the affluent becomes available to those lower down the social scale with whatever pathogenic influences for anorexia nervosa that it may contain.

Familial Factors in Anorexia nervosa

THEANDER calculated from his material that a sister of a patient with anorexia nervosa has a morbidity risk of 6.6% (±2.4%) which is way above the most generous estimate of the prevalence of the illness. A family in which a mother and daughter had the illness is described by CRISP [1965], and THEANDER mentions a case of a mother and two daughters all with anorexia nervosa but not from his own series.

CRISP and TOMS [1972] describe a remarkable family in which a male with anorexia nervosa had an adopted daughter who herself developed anorexia nervosa. Another girl who had spent a period living with this family during the war, also developed anorexia nervosa at a later date. In the CRISP and TOMS series of male anorexics there is a high incidence of anorexia nervosa in siblings with one patient having an affected brother and two, an affected sister.

Twin Studies

There has been a number of twin studies published containing both concordant and discordant pairs of identical twins, some with a minimum of clinical description and, at the other extreme, the very detailed study of GIFFORD *et al,* [1970] of a discordant pair of twins. A drawback of some of the published discordant pairs is that the unaffected twin has still to live through the total period of risk, for example case 2 of HALMI and BRODLAND [1973] where the twins were aged 12 at time of publication. Their other cases of concordant twins is of great interest in this respect as the second twin did not develop anorexia nervosa until the age of 38, shortly after the death of her sister. This case highlights another of the difficulties of interpreting twin studies, namely that the forces of identification, often so powerful in identical twins, are likely to overshadow any effect that may be due to common genetic endowment. Thus, although the classical approach to twin studies of comparing concordance rates in identical and fraternal twins, derived in some consistent fashion from the population, has not yet been applied to anorexia nervosa, even an increased incidence of concordance in identical twins would not be absolute evidence for a genetic determination.

Of the published studies, discordant pairs are described by KOLUCH and DAVIDOVA [1962]; CRISP [1966] (one personal case and two others communicated to him); BRUCH [1969] (two cases plus one other communicated to her); GIFFORD *et al.* [1970]; MORMONT and DEMOULIN [1971]; HALMI and BRODLAND [1973]; in all ten pairs. Concordant pairs are recorded by BOM [1940], DÜHRSSEN [1950], MEYER [1961], ZIOLKO [1966], THEANDER [1970] (not a personal case), HALMI and BRODLAND [1973], in all 6 cases. In view of the lack of differentiation of aetiological factors in concordant twins it is probably more profitable to study discordant twin pairs. HALMI and BRODLAND [1973] report a twin who developed anorexia nervosa when aged 10½ following a fever that produced a rapid loss of 2.5 kg. The patient had been the heavier at birth. There was no clear dominance in the relationship, both were somewhat neurotic. The patient recovered her pre morbid weight. Both twins were 12 and still pre-menarchic at the time of publication. In their very ample study, GIFFORD *et al.* [1970] make the general observation that already at birth there are considerable intra-pair differences, particularly in nutritional status. The affected twin had always weighed less and had been more difficult to feed as an infant. The unaffected twin was very much the leader of the two and was generally more assertive and forthright and more interested in boyfriends. The unaffected twin became pregnant at age 18, while the patient's amenorrhoea commenced just after the sister's baby was born. Also, at this time the patient was forced to go to a distant college and a brother committed suicide. Over the subsequent year the patient was very unhappy and gained some weight, but thereafter began losing much weight which coincided with her sister's engagement and the breaking off of her own engagement. With treatment she regained some weight but did not make substantial improvement until her sister broke off her engagement. The picture that emerged of the patient's differential vulnerability were her pre-morbid passivity, the nutritional difficulties and the threat that separation and her sister's sexual activity presented. However, it would be an over-simplification to dismiss the brother's suicide and the father's depressive illness as traumas common to the two sisters and therefore irrelevant, as it is likely that the relationship meant more to the affected sister in some degree due to her more withdrawn personality and the greater difficulty that she had in making relationships outside the family.

BRUCH [1969] described two discordant pairs. In the first, the patient weighed slightly less than her sister at birth and was less eager at the breast. Thoughout childhood she was regarded as less attractive in temperament than the other. The healthy twin was very definitely the leader and although interested in remaining slim she maintained her slimness in a fairly normal fashion. The patient was more prone to overeat and vomit. When her sister's engagement was announced the patient became depressed and grossly underweight. With treatment she improved greatly.

In the other set of twins, the patient was 4.5 lb. at birth and her sister was 7 lb., always remaining the heavier one thereafter. The patient's menarche came 1 month later than her sister's when aged 13. The mother was always concerned about the patient's undernourished look as a child although the twins both became overweight in adolescence. At college the sister led an active social life and the patient's self-starvation began.

CRISP [1966] described a discordant pair in detail. The patient was slightly heavier than her sister at birth and was always regarded as the submissive one, shy and 'pretty highly strung'. Her periods commenced at 14.5 years and those of her sister at 12.5 years. The parents' marriage was unstable and the patient felt far more involved and concerned about this than her sister. The patient had more difficulty in relating to boyfriends than did her sister and the illness began at the time of her sister's engagement. CRISP [1966] gives limited description of two other pairs known to two other psychiatrists. In both pairs the affected sister was considered less mature and more submissive in the twinship.

MORMONT and DEMOULIN [1971] have described a pair of identical twins discordant for anorexia nervosa in which the healthy one was clearly dominant, protecting the patient at school. When the patient was aged 17 her mother nade her terminate a platonic affair with a boyfriend and she became uninterested in men thereafter. Her sister became engaged and it was at about this time that the patient developed anorexia nervosa.

The picture that emerges from these studies is of the submissive, more generally dependant twin reacting to the rupture of the twinship due to the engagement or some other activity of her sister, with the emergence of anorexia nervosa. There is no clear evidence from this small series of why the twin developed anorexia nervosa rather than some other reaction. There is some suggestion that the affected twin had some nutritional disadvantage from birth or even *in utero*. It is a pity that the twins concordant for anorexia nervosa are generally less well descirbed than the dicordant pairs but there are some features wothy of note. The Halmi and Brodland pair are very unusual, with the late onset of disease at 37 of the second sister, following the death of the first. In both the Ziolko and the Meyer pairs there is a very disparate development after the illness in each twin. In the Ziolko pair, one became alcoholic with multiple suicidal attempts while the other entered into a useful psychotherapeutic relationship. In the Meyer pair, despite a remarkable coincidence of onset and termination of the illness, the one twin became completely well, married and had children while the other stayed at home and developed what was judged to be a chronic schizophrenic illness. We can conclude from the weight of discordant studies that the vicissitudes of human development, possibly beginning even *in utero,* have a major bearing on whether the individual develops anorexia nervosa. This is not to say that genetic factors are of no importance. It seems likely that the anorexia nervosa patient has a special type of metabolism that allows her to lose so much weight and still remain energetic and capable. In other more primitive circumstances the behaviour could be highly adaptive and allow the individual to survive a period of famine. In this context it is of interest to note that most anorexics are at some time obese, demonstrating the parallel capacity to store food at times of plenty.

THEANDER [1970] reports 50% of patients describing themselves as overweight premorbidly and HALMI [1974] gives a figure of 38% who were 7 kg or more above the weight given for their height on standard tables.

Anorexia nervosa and Gonadal Dysgenesis

A number of studies have appeared in which the concurrence of anorexia nervosa with gonadal dysgenesis has been reported by PITTS and GUZE [1963], FORSSMAN *et al.* [1970], DICKENS [1970], HALMI and RIGAS [1973]. (The cases reported by LINDSTEN [1963] and KIHLBOM [1969] are diagnostically uncertain.) It is difficult to know whether this is more than a chance association. The prevalence of gonadal dysgenesis is approximately 1:3,000 females but the true prevalence of anorexia nervosa is uncertain.

LISTON and SHERSHOW [1973] have made a very rough calculation, given 17.2 million females in the USA who had entered or passed through the second decade of life between 1960 and 1970. Taking a prevalence for anorexia nervosa of 50–75/100,000 females at risk, there should have been 10,000 females with anorexia nervosa during this time. With a rate for gonadal dysgenesis of 1:3,000, this should have by chance produced 3 cases in the USA during this time. Only 2 have been reported. It seems essentially unlikely that all examples of the association have been both observed and reported but at the moment the case must remain open. Although a rarity, it would be very important for our more complete understanding of the psychopathology and constitutional background of anorexia nervosa if the association were confirmed. HALMI and RIGAS [1973] have claimed an association between urogenital malformations generally and anorexia nervosa. They advance the hypothesis, that there is a genetic linkage between gonadal dysgenesis and anorexia nervosa; simple urogenital malformations may be due to mosaicism in which the chromosomal abnormality is localised in the cells of the urogenital system.

Anorexia nervosa and Pregnancy

Anorexia nervosa has been recorded in pregnancy. LAKOFF and FELDMAN [1972] record a case and mention two others. In their own patient, the marriage had been precipitated by the pregnancy. The patient was delivered at 40 weeks of a girl weighing 4 lb. 13 oz. The baby was considered a small, full-term one, rather than premature. There was no obvious developmental retardation. The patient recovered her normal weight soon after delivery.

Although an individual with a potential for anorexia nervosa would avoid pregnancy, if she should achieve pregnancy this would seem likely to constitute a very major stress. From the rarity of the reports it would seem likely that the potential anorexic is very well defended against becoming pregnant until she is ready for it. On the other hand, it may be that a re-evaluation of hyperemesis gravidarum may reveal that it is a congener of anorexia nervosa.

Pre-Morbid Factors Associated with Anorexia nervosa

RUSSELL [1972] has taken a group of 231 nurses, medical students and school girls and has ascertained that 15% have at one time lost 7 lb. or more in weight, 6% have had secondary amenorrhoea of at least 6 months duration and 4% reported a combination of the two anomalies. Clearly he was not dealing with anorexia nervosa as commonly defined but his further findings are likely to be germane to the illness. He investigated a group of 25 patients with established anorexia nervosa using the above population as his control group and established that in this group of patients there was a significant excess of second born children and less contact with grandparents particularly the maternal grandmother. There was a significant increase in the number of maternal grandmothers who had died by the patients' tenth birthday, usually during the patients' early childhood. There was a strong trend for the patients to have come from social class I or II, to have had a boarding school, education and to have had three or more moves of home. There was a significant correlation between the number of these experiences and the severity of the loss in weight.

He then ascertained the correlation between these factors and loss of weight and amenorrhoea in the control group and found that in the weight loss group 40% had been exposed to three or more of the above experiences as against only 23% in the remainder of the group. For amenorrhoea the figures were similarly 57% against 23% ($p<0.02$). In the group with both symptoms the difference was greatest, 66 versus 24% ($p=0.02$). Examined from another angle, of the 44 girls who had none of these experiences only 1 had weight loss and amenorrhoea. Of the 59 girls who had 3 or more experiences, 6 had weight loss and amenorrhoea. This data strenghens the case that even fairly minor episodes of weight loss and amenorrhoea may belong to the same psychopathological continuum as anorexia nervosa.

Some of these specific items have been pursued by other authors. There is general agreement that anorexia nervosa patients tend to come from the upper and middle classes, but uncertainty about whether this was a feature of the illness or of the greater likelihood of medical attention. RUSSELL's finding would tend to favour the former. In THEANDER's [1970] group of 94 patients there is a well-marked excess of second born patients (30 versus 21 first born, from sibships of 2 or more), but the difference does not achieve statistical significance. CRISP [1970] shows a similar trend in his series (22 versus 17). CRISP [1970] has produced carefully controlled data on birth weight and menarche in a group of anorexia nervosa patients, that although there was no difference in birth weight when compared to matched controls, he found that when compared to their sisters the patients were 13 oz. heavier at birth – a highly significant difference ($p<0.005$). Although most of the variance was contributed by the segment of the patient group that had been born later than the control sister, there was nonetheless a strong trend, albeit short of statistical significance, in the other segment of patients born earlier than their control sister.

The age of menarche was not different when compared to their sisters but was significantly younger than a matched control population (12 years 8 months versus 13 years 6 months; $p<0.003$).

THEANDER [1970] finds in his study that the maternal age at the birth of the patient is significantly higher than the national average and the finding is not due simply to the patients' being born later into the sibship. HALMI [1974] confirms the observation and extends it to paternal age as well. It is possible that this datum is linked to social class difference.

Conclusion

We can conclude that there is a wide spectrum of disorder characterised by loss of weight and amenorrhoea which at its simplest level may be shown at some time by at least 4% of the female teen-age population. The 'true' incidence of 'clinical anorexia nervosa' is unknown but it is being seen with increasing frequency by doctors.

Recent yearly incidences are in the range of 3–14 cases for 100,000 women in the 15–34 age group. The lifetime risk is likely to be of the order of 6 times the yearly incidence. There is no data on the extent to which equally severe cases are never identified by doctors but they are likely to constitute a substantial population.

Pre-morbidly, patients are more likely to be born into the upper social classes, to be overweight, have a sister with anorexia nervosa, to be the submissive in a pair of identical twins, or to be the second born in a normal sibship. The illness has been described in most of the countries of Europe, the USA and Japan. Until adequate surveys have been carried out it will not be possible to know whether the illness is found only in food-rich cultures.

The clinical description of the illness in males are very similar to those described in the female. The relative incidence is likely to lie between 1:4 and 1:15 with an earlier manifestation of the illness in the male. There is a considerable need for true epidemiological studies of anorexia nervosa in the community and cross-cultural comparisons.

References

BEUMONT, P.J.V.; BEARDWOOD, C.J., and RUSSELL G.F.M.: The occurrence of the syndrome of anorexia nervosa in male subjects. Psychol. Med. *2:* 216–231 (1972).

Bom, F.: Simmond's syndrom (endogen afmagring) hos et par enaeggede tvillinger. Nord. Med. *8:* 2506–2510 (1940).

Bruch, H.: The psychiatric differential diagnosis of anorexia nervosa; in Meyer and Feldmann Anorexia nervosa. Symposium Göttingen (Stuttgart 1965).

Bruch, H.: Anorexia nervosa and its differential diagnosis. J. nerv. ment. Dis. *141:* 555 (1966).

Bruch, H.: The insignificant difference: discordant incidence of anorexia nervosa in monozygotic twins. Am. J. Psychiat. *126:* 85–90 (1969).

Bruch, H.: Anorexia nervosa in the male. Psychosom. Med. *33:* 31–47 (1971).

Crisp, A.H.: Clinical and therapeutic aspects of anorexia nervosa. A study of 30 cases. J. psychosom. Res. *9:* 67–78 (1965).

Crisp, A.H.: Anorexia nervosa in identical twins. Postgrad. med. J. *42:* 86 (1966).

Crisp. A.H.: Reported birth weights and growth rates in a group of patients with primary anorexia nervosa (weight phobia). J. psychosom. Res. *14:* 23–50 (1970).

Crisp, A.H. and Toms, D.A.: Primary anorexia nervosa or weight phobia in the male. Report on 13 cases. Br. med. J. *1:* 334–338 (1972).

Dickens, J.A.: Concurrence of Turner's syndrome and anorexia nervosa. Br. J. Psychiat. *117:* 237 (1970).

Dührssen, A.: Zum Problem der psychogenen Ess-Störung. Psyche *4:* 56 (1950).

Feighner, J.P.; Robins, E.; Guze, S.B.; Woodruff, R.A., jr.; Winokur, G., and Munoz, R.: Diagnostic criteria for use in psychiatric research. Archs. gen. Psychiat. *26:* 57–63 (1972).

Forssman, H.; Mellbin, G., and Walinder, J.: Concurrence of Turner's syndrome and anorexia nervosa. Br. J. Psychiat. *116:* 221–223 (1970).

Gifford, S.; Murawski, B.J., and Pilot, M.L.: Anorexia nervosa in one of identical twins. Int. psychiat. Clin. *7:* 139–228 (1970).

Halmi, K.A.: Anorexia nervosa. Demographic and clinical features in 94 cases. Psychosom. Med. *36:* 18–26 (1974).

Halmi, K. and Brodland, G.: Monozygotic twins concordant and discordant for anorexia nervosa. Psychol. Med. *3:* 521–524 (1973).

Halmi, K.A. and Rigas, C.: Urogenital malformations associated with anorexia nervosa. Br. J. Psychiat. *122:* 79–81 (1973).

Kay, D.W.K. and Schapira, K.: Psychiatric observations on anorexia; in Reichsman Hunger and satiety in health and disease (Karger, Basel 1972).

Kendell, R.E.; Hall, D.J.; Hailey, A., and Babigan, H.M.: The epidemiology of anorexia nervosa. Psychol. Med. *3:* 200–203 (1973).

Kilbom, M.: Psychopathology of Turner's syndrome. Acta paedospychiat. *36:* 75–81 (1969)

Koluch, J. und Davidova, M.: Zur Problematik der Anorexia mentalis. Acta paedopsychiat. *29:* 343–349 (1962).

Lakoff, K.M. and Feldman, J.D.: Anorexia nervosa associated with pregnancy. Obstet. Gynec. *39:* 699 (1972).

Lindsten, J.. The nature and origin of X chromosome observation in Turner's syndrome (Almqvist & Wiksell, Stockholm 1973).

Lipowski, Z.J.: Psychosocial aspects of physical illness (Karger, Basel 1972).

Liston, E.H. and Shershow, L.W.: Concurrence of anorexia nervosa and gonadal dysgenesis (Turner's syndrome). Archs. gen. Psychiat. *29:* 834 (1973).

MEYER, J.E.: Das Syndrom der Anorexia nervosa. Arch. Psychiat. Nerv. Krankh. *202:* 31–59 (1961).

MORGAN, G. and SYLVESTER, D.G.H.: Personal commun. (1974).

MORMONT, C. and DEMOULIN, C.: Personality of a mental anorexia patient and of her monozygotic twin. Acta psychiat. belg. *71:* 477–487 (1971).

PITTS, F.N. and GUZE, S.B.: Anorexia nervosa and gonadal dysgenesis (Turner's syndrome). Am. J. Psychiat. *119:* 1100–1102 (1963).

ROWLAND, C.V.: Anorexia nervosa. A survey of the literature and review of 30 cases. Int. psychiat. Clin. *7:* 37–137 (1970).

RUSSELL, J.A.O.: Psychosocial aspects of weight loss and amenorrhoea in adolescent girls; in MORRIS Psychosomatic medicine in obstetrics and gynaecology (Karger, Basel 1972).

SEAVER, R.L. and BINDER, H.J.: Anorexia nervosa and other anorectic states in man; in REICHSMAN Hunger and satiety in health and disease (Karger, Basel 1972).

SELVINI, P.M.: Interpretation of mental anorexia; in MEYER and FELDMANN, Anorexia nervosa. Symposium Göttingen (Stuttgart 1965).

THEANDER, S.: Anorexia nervosa. Acta psychiat. scand., suppl. 214 (1970).

THOMA, H.: Treatment of anorexia nervosa; in REICHSMAN Hunger and satiety in health and disease (Karger, Basel 1972).

ZIOLKO, H.U.: Anorexia nervosa. Fortsch. Neurol. Psychiat. *34:* 353–396 (1966).

Dr. O.W. HILL, Department of Psychiatry, Middlesex Hospital, *London W 1N8 AA* (England)

Adv. psychosom. Med., vol. 9, pp. 63–104 (Karger, Basel 1977)

The Effects of Bereavement and Grief on Physical Health and General Well-Being

GERALD L. KLERMAN and JUDITH E. IZEN

Harvard Medical School and Psychiatric Service, Massachusetts General Hospital, Boston, Mass.

Contents

Introduction

Purpose

From the beginning of recorded history, grief and mourning have been recognized as being capable of producing bodily changes in the bereaved. Isaiah, in biblical times, admonished his fellow Israelites to 'Bind up the Broken Hearted' and the literature from other cultures and eras have also noted the physical effects of grief. In recent years, there has been an explosion of scientific interest in the impact of grief, loss, and separation upon social functioning, psychiatric illness and personal health. Considerable research has been done on the phenomena of grief itself and also upon the consequences of loss and grief for the individual as manifested by susceptibility to illness in general and to psychiatric disorders, such as depression.

This paper will review and evaluate the evidence in support of the proposition that individuals experiencing loss are susceptible to medical illnesses, impairment of their general well-being and even increase in mortality. This paper will not review the grief syndrome itself because of the extensive literature available on the subject elsewhere, i.e., ENGEL [1961] and FREUD [1917] although we will touch upon it in passing. Nor will we discuss the important relationships between loss and various psychiatric illness, particularly depression, as demonstrated in various studies, i.e., PARKES [1964], PAYKEL *et al.* [1969] and SETHI [1964]. Rather we shall focus on general health as manifested by mortality, specific medical illnesses, and general well-being. Following the review and evaluation of the evidence, we shall discuss the possible mechanisms by which loss and resultant grief could alter susceptibility to illness. We shall then explore the implications of these processes for human adaptation.

Loss, Bereavement and Grief

The terms 'bereavement' and 'grief' are usually used synonymously. However, we feel it is important to distinguish bereavement – the objective situation of an individual having lost a significant person by death from grief – the bodily, emotional and psychological changes that the bereaved individual usually, but not always, expresses. Although most individuals who are bereaved manifest grief, there are important exceptions. As LINDEMANN [1945] observed, some bereaved individuals have delayed grief or never grieve at all. Based on this observation, a number of hypotheses have been formulated predicting that individuals who do not grieve, or whose grief is delayed or in some sense atypical are susceptible to psychosomatic illness.

To avoid confusion we shall utilize the following terminology: bereavement shall refer to the objective state of an individual who has experienced loss by death of a significant person, usually a spouse, parent, child, other family member, or close friend. Grief shall refer to the complex of bodily, emotional, cognitive, and psychosocial changes manifested in response to the bereavement.

Most current research on grief follows the pioneering studies of LINDEMANN. In 1945, LINDEMANN observed the manifestations of grief in a large group of individuals who were bereaved in the Cocanut Grove fire.

He described the stages of normal grief as involving: (a) initial shock; (b) intense affects of sadness; (c) withdrawal from the environment; (d) protest of the loss, and then (e) a gradual resolution of the grief. LINDEMANN concluded that the 'normal' bereaved individual took about a year to 'work through' his/her grief.

LINDEMANN identified five characteristics that were 'pathognomic' of abnormal or atypical grief reactions. These pathognomic qualities of 'abnormal' grief were: somatic distress, preoccupation with the deceased, feelings of guilt, loss of warmth in relationships with other people, and a disorganized pattern of conduct. Based upon his clinical observations of 'pathognomic' varients of grief, LINDEMANN hypothesized that the inability to grieve normally following loss results in a greater susceptibility to psychosomatic illness. Furthermore, he postulated that serious difficulties could result from an inability to grieve after bereavement due to the repression or alteration of 'normal' grief process.

Building upon LINDEMANN's work, ENGEL in his 1964 paper, 'Is Grief a Disease', reviewed the empirical studies of the grieving state and concluded that normal grief should be considered a disease state brought about by object loss. ENGEL proposed that grief was a well-defined clinical syndrome with specific symptoms, following a predictable course leading to recovery in the majority of instances. However, he noted that there were 'complicated outcomes' resulting from internal psychic structure which may delay or prolong grief or which may result in unusual physical or psychological manifestations in the grief state.

In the decade since ENGEL's classic paper, a considerable literature has developed upon the diverse aspects of the grieving state. The interested reader is referred to the excellent reports by CLAYTON [1968], PARKES [1970] and MADDISON and VIOLA [1968] among others. The thrust of their research has been to verify most of the hypotheses formulated by LINDEMANN and ENGEL and to document the complex and diverse nature of the grief state and its variations. These studies also report the sequence of events in grief over time leading to recovery or residual impairments and/or heightened susceptibility to illness.

Although most of the interest in loss has centered around the 'objective' bereavement that follows death of a loved one, there is an important body of thinking that has extended the concept of loss to include anticipated threat of loss or psychological meanings given to events other than death of a loved one. The point of view expressed in this approach is that the psychological meaning of an event as a 'loss' is more important than whether or not there has been an actual loss.

This approach is best represented by the Rochester group, particularly by the writings of ENGEL, GREENE and SCHMALE. SCHMALE [1958] found that 98% of the patients admitted to a general hospital experienced a loss of an object which was accompanied by feelings of helplessness and hopelessness prior to the onset of their disease. There were 42 patients in the sample and the average age was 31. There was no control group in this study. The definition of loss in this study was very broad including actual loss, actual threat of loss, and symbolic loss of an object. *Actual* loss of an object was experienced by 12% (5) of the 42 patients. These losses included death of a sibling, broken engagement, marital separation, etc. 21% (9) of the patients had experienced *actual threat* of a loss such as change of health, negative change in the behavior of a significant other, etc. 38% (16 subjects) had experienced *symbolic loss* of an object such as failing grades, friend forgetting a date, etc. 29% (12) of the patients reported no loss of a significant other although SCHMALE was able to make an 'interpretation' of actual, threatened, or symbolic loss for 11 out of the 12 patients. The interval between the final feelings of hopelessness and helplessness and the onset of the disease was within 25 h for 38% (16 patients) and within 1 week for 36% (15 patients). The patients suffered from a diverse group of diseases, the majority of them being cardiovascular (17%), diseases of the nervous system (17%), digestive (12%), respiratory (12%), and other disease groups.

SCHMALE's paper is one of the most oft-quoted in the field but it presents a problem in theory and methodology. His categories of 'object loss' are very broad and include almost every event that could occur to a 'normal' individual in the course of a lifetime. This fact points out the need for a control group to determine whether the hospitalized population did indeed experience a higher degree of object loss. Another methodological problem is that SCHMALE did not separate death of a significant other from the category of 'actual losses of objects'. This prevents comparison with other studies that do separate death of a significant other from other losses.

A significant finding in SCHMALE's study, however, is his report of feelings of helplessness and hopelessness in the hospitalized patients. The cause and effect mechanism of hopelessness and disease is not known. The causal relationship could be that either the disease causes the feelings of helplessness and hopelessness or that the feelings of helplessness and hopelessness (due presumably to the object loss) are a precipitant to the onset of disease. SCHMALE takes the position that the feelings of helplessness and hopelessness are an important factor in the etiology of the disease.

A theoretical problem in SCHMALE's paper is his inclusion of 'symbolic loss' or 'fantasied loss' in addition to the category of 'actual loss' of object. There has been some dispute in the field concerning this practice although STOECKLE and DAVIDSON [1962] point out that sometimes the fantasied losses were more traumatic to the subjects than an actual loss would have been. It is too soon to evaluate the full significance of this approach which attempts to extend the concept of loss to include 'fantasied loss'. Its potential benefit would be to draw attention to the psychological meaning which individuals give to events, particularly the psychological attitudes around helplessness and hopelessness as intervening processes between the actual objective loss and the psychosomatic impact upon the individual.

For the purposes of this paper, however, we shall focus predominantly on those studies which have dealt with actual loss through bereavement of a significant other. We will not deal with the bereavement due to loss of a body part such as limb, loss of home, occupation or job, or other losses. In doing so we are choosing bereavement due to death of a significant other as the 'extreme case'. Bereavement due to loss of a significant other represents the purest form of the loss paradigm and as such should be the natural situation most amenable to research analysis.

Life Stress

Before discussing the evidence relating bereavement and grief to mortality and specific illnesses, it is desirable to relate the grief and bereavement process to the more general psychobiological processes concerned with life change and environmental stress. Following upon the teachings of MEYER [1948] many psychiatrists have identified environmental factors as precipitants for various types of illness and emphasized the role of changes in life events as part of the total adjustment of the individual. The psychosomatic movement of the 1930s and 1940s produced a number of important clinical and research approaches, most particularly those of ALEXANDER [1939], COBB and LINDEMANN [1943] and WOLFF [1953]. These efforts generated a number of imaginative hypotheses concerning relationships between life stress and environmental events in general; loss, bereavement and grief in particular; in the predisposition to or precipitation of a variety of psychiatric and medical illnesses. Research on loss and grief is a subset of general stress theory. Loss through bereavement is a special case of stress to which the individual must adapt.

It is only in the past two decades that these general ideas have been defined with sufficient precision to be subjected to verification by empirical studies employing modern research design, quantitative techniques and advanced statistical methods. The most significant advances in this research field have followed from the work of HOLMES and RAHE [1967] who developed a quantitative technique for assessing various types of life events including loss and bereavement. Their 'Social Readjustment Rating Scale' (SRRS) quantitatively assesses the frequency and magnitude of recent changes in a person's environment. Loss of a spouse is considered the most severe life change and is weighted the most heavily; other severe changes, such as sickness of relatives, moving or loss of a job are weighted less heavily. Studies of 'normal' and physically sick populations demonstrate a higher incidence of change and loss in the lives of persons in the months preceeding onset of various illnesses [RAHE and ARTHUR, 1968]. The scale also asks subjects to subjectively determine their response to each life change and their response to the stress [HOLMES and RAHE, 1967]. The scale is used extensively by clinicians and researchers studying 'life events' and onset of physical and mental illness [GRANT *et al.,* 1974; HUDGENS *et al.,* 1967; MYERS *et al.,* 1971].

The findings from these studies have generally supported the proposition that life stress, of all sorts, places individuals at 'greater risk', i.e. more susceptible to, a variety of physical illnesses and psychiatric states. Viewed in this context, loss through bereavement would represent one specific aspect of a life event and stress. Obviously, there will be a major overlap in research findings and theoretical conceptualizations between life stress research and loss and bereavement research. At some point in the future it will be necessary to separate out those processes which are specific to loss through bereavement and those which are part of a general stress and adaptation response in the individual.

To anticipate some of the conclusions from this future research, our point of view is that the reactions of loss due to bereavement activate the very powerful psychobiological mechanisms associated with attachment bonding. The disruption of this bond initiates very intense emotional and biological events which have a physiological basis in mammalian evolutionary history. The stress response, particularly those mediated by the neuroendocrine system, is one of the systems activated by the disruption of attachment bonding. It is our view that the attachment bonding mechanisms are stimulus-specific and more intense in many of their manifestations than the general stress response. However, these thoughts are at this moment speculative and require further research for verification.

Epidemiologic Focus

In view of the vact that the focus of this volume is upon epidemiologic studies, it is incumbent upon us to translate these research and clinical trends into an epidemiologic perspective. Epidemiology is concerned with the rates of occurrence of illness within a population and the factors which render certain individuals 'at risk' for illness.

Translating the previously mentioned clinical hypotheses into epidemiologic language, the general proposition would state that individuals who experience loss via bereavement constitute a population greater 'at risk' for physical illness.

A corollary of this general proposition would include predictions of an increase in: (1) general mortality rate; (2) onset and incidence of a number of specific disorders, such as cardiovascular, cancer, and the so-called 'psychosomatic' disorders; (3) increase in death by suicide, and (4) increase in various forms of health-care seeking behavior.

A related set of hypotheses predict that among the bereaved, those who fail to grieve are at even greater risk for illness in general and especially for the subgroup of the so-called 'psychosomatic' illnesses in particular.

In order to verify these hypotheses, not only are clinical survey techniques needed but also available knowledge such as base rates in comparable populations matched for age, sex, social class, race and other relevant demographic characteristics.

The crucial methodological issue for epidemiologic studies is the capacity to calculate rates and to compare rates between populations. Two general methods have been employed in conducting this type of research: those using historical base rates and those using concurrent control groups.

Studies using historical, or baseline, rates rely upon previously conducted research in the hopes that they will have generated established norms. For example, several studies have attempted to determine 'the normal loss rates' within a population [IMBODEN *et al.* 1963; MURPHY, 1962]. IMBODEN *et al.* [1963] determined the 'normal bereavement rates' of a normal population of 455 men (employees at an army fort, average age 35). The authors report that 25.7% of the men reported *some* type of separation from family members (such as spouse, parent, or close relative) in the form of divorce, marital separation, or death or illness of relative within 1 year of the index date. 8.9% of these losses were of *death* of a family member within 1 year of the index date. The authors note that the group that experienced losses (25.7% of the men) did not visit the dispensary for symptomatic complaints over an 18-month period more than the group that did not experience any losses. In a study on a female population hospitalized for normal delivery, approximately 35% of women experienced *sickness or death* in their family in the 1-year prior to their admission. Less than 30% of the women experienced what the authors term 'disturbed interpersonal relationships' during the same time period [MURPHY, 1962].

Theses studies give us some baseline rates of loss or threat of loss of a significant other in a 1-year period for a 'normal' population. These rates (approximately 25% for some loss or threat of loss and around 8.9% for death of a significant other) for a 'normal' population can be compared to the rates of bereavemement in a 'sick' population. The Imboden and Murphy studies can serve as some basis of comparison to determine if the studies that find a 'sick' population experiencing a high incidence of bereavement are actually finding a significant variable or a 'normal' rate of bereavement.

The historical studies are valuable in giving certain general estimates as to the rates of loss and related events in a 'normal' population but from the methodological point of view they cannot be as powerful as the use of concurrent controls. As we will discuss later in this chapter, the most powerful evidence for the impact of loss comes from those studies which have matched a population 'at risk' with a concurrent control group. Various problems in sampling, population characteristics such as age, sex, race, etc., and historical events such as epidemics, nutritional status, etc., are always operative to render imprecise the extrapolations from base rates calculated from previous reports regardless of how well they were conducted. For these reasons, in the body of this paper we shall give greater weight to those studies which rely upon concurrent controls for calculation of rates even though we recognize that other forms of baseline comparisons are of value.

Sources of Evidence

Having reviewed these general considerations of our hypothesis with regard to overall theory and methodology for epidemiologic studies, we are now in a position to initiate a systematic review of the sources of evidence relative to the relationship between bereavement and grief on the physical health and general well-being in individuals experiencing loss.

The next sections of this paper will review in detail the sources of evidence in a number of areas. These are: (1) increase in general mortality rates; (2) suicide; (3) specific medical disorders; (4) decrease in general well-being; and (5) increase in health-care seeking behavior.

Increase in Overall Mortality Rates

Evidence for Increased Mortality

The most powerful impact of bereavement and grief would be upon overall mortality. If it could be demonstrated with some certainty that the bereaved are truly at 'greater risk' for mortality, the importance of bereavement and grief would be clearly established. The search for possible mechanisms, physiological and psychsosmatic, would than be placed upon a very firm foundation. Therefore, the most important source of evidence is

Table I. Mortality ratios for widowed males and females compared to married males and females (white and nonwhite, age 20–44)

	Males			Females		
	20–24	25–34	35–44	20–24	25–34	35–44
White	3.87	4.31	2.88	3.70	2.66	1.83
Nonwhite	2.58	3.88	2.94	2.27	2.37	1.92

From KRAUS and LILIENFELD [1959].

from those studies which claim to demonstrate an increase in overall mortality among those individuals who have been recently bereaved.

KRAUS and LILIENFELD [1959] reported one of the earliest studies on the subject of mortality in the bereaved. They retrospectively calculated mortality rates for widows and widowers matching data from the National Office of Vital Statistics for the year 1956 with the data from the 1950 census. Death rates of widowed subjects were compared to the rates for married men and women matched for age, sex and race. These data are summarized in table I. The death rate for white widowers, age 25–34, was 4.3 times greater than the death rate for white married males of the same age. For nonwhite widowers, age 25–34 years, the mortality rate was 3.9 times greater than married controls. White widows, age 25–34 years, had a mortality rate 2.7 times greater than white married females and nonwhite widows from the same age group had a mortality rate 2.8 times greater than their controls. The mortality ratio of widowed to married decreased as the age increased for both sexes and races. Specifically, younger widows and widowers (ages 20–24 and 25–34 years) compared to the young married group had the highest ratio of mortality for eight causes of death including: vascular lesions of the central nervous system (ratio for age 20–24 widows was 11.7 times greater than their married controls), arteriosclerotic heart disease (rate was 14.4 times greater for widows age 20–24), nonrheumatic chronic endocarditis and other myocardial degeneration (rate was 12.7 times higher for widowers age 24–35 compared to their matched controls), hypertension with heart disease (rate was 18.4 times greater for widows age 20–24), general arteriosclerosis (the mortality rate for widows age 24–34 was 36.7 times higher than married controls), tuberculosis (rate was 12.7 times higher for widowers age 24–34 than for married men of the same age), and influenza and pneu-

Table II. Average annual death ratio for selected causes for age 20–44 group, by age and sex (United States 1949–1951)

	Widowed rate divided by married rate by age					
	Males			Females		
	20–24	24–34	35–44	20–24	24–34	35–44
Vascular lesions of CNS	11.7	8.1	4.0	6.2	4.2	2.9
Disease of the heart	7.8	5.1	2.5	5.6	3.8	2.8
Arteriosclerotic heart disease	–	4.9	2.0	1.4	5.9	2.7
Nonrheumatic chronic endo-carditis and other myocardial degeneration	–	12.7	4.3	11.3	6.5	3.9
Hypertension with heart disease	–	10.8	4.6	18.4	4.7	3.6
General arterio-sclerosis	–	–	–	–	36.7	6.5
Tuberculosis	8.1	12.7	7.7	5.7	4.9	3.4
Influenza and pneumonia	–	7.7	6.7	4.2	5.0	3.9
Malignant neoplasms	–	2.3	2.1	2.4	2.5	1.8
of digestive organs and peritoneum	–	4.0	2.4	–	2.8	1.9
of respiratory system	–	5.0	2.2	–	–	–
of breast	–	–	–	–	1.9	1.3
of genital organs	–	–	–	4.1	3.4	2.4
Diabetes	–	3.3	2.5	–	2.5	2.9
Chronic and unspecified nephritis and other renal sclerosis	–	2.6	3.2	–	2.8	2.5
Cirrhosis of the liver	–	5.6	4.1	–	–	–
Motor vehicle accidents	3.1	4.5	3.2	0.9	3.3	2.6
All other accidents	2.4	3.1	3.0	4.4	3.9	2.8
Suicide	9.3	6.9	3.5	–	–	–

Extrapolated from table III in KRAUS and LILIENFELD [1959].

monia (the mortality rate was 7.7 times higher for widowers age 24–34 than for matched married males). These data can be seen in table II.

When all of these disease groups were combined, the mortality rate was at least 7 times greater among the young widowed group (under age 45 years) than for the matched young married control group. The young male widowers were especially at 'high risk' for death from cardiovascular disease in which the mortality rate for the young widowers was 10 times higher than for the married men of the same age. KRAUS and LILIENFELD concluded that as a group, the recently bereaved were greater 'at risk' for mortality.

REES and LUTKINS [1967] in a prospective study followed a cohort of 903 relatives of 371 residents of a village in Wales who had died during the previous year. These 903 bereaved relatives were compared to a cohort of 878 nonbereaved family members who were matched as to age, sex, and marital status with the deceased. These cohorts were followed for 6 years. The mortality rate for the bereaved spouses was significantly greater than for the control spouses – 12% of bereaved spouses died during the 1st year of bereavement compared to 1% of nonbereaved spouses (significant at the $p=0.01$ level). 7% of bereaved spouses died during the 2nd year, compared to 3% of nonbereaved control spouses, and 3% of bereaved spouses died during the 3rd year of bereavement compared to 2% of nonbereaved spouses. The mortality rate of bereaved spouses is not significantly different for the 2nd and 3rd year than the rate of the controls.

The mortality rate of other bereaved close relatives (parents, children, and siblings) was also significant when compared to the control group of nonbereaved relatives. 3.2% of the bereaved relatives died within 1 year compared to 0.6% of the controls. This death rate is 6 times greater (significant at the $p=0.001$ level). During the 2nd year of bereavement the difference in mortality rates was not significant – 2.0% of bereaved relatives died compared to 1.3% of nonbereaved control relatvies. There was also no significant difference in mortality in the 3rd year of bereavement. In general, the death rate increase was greatest for male relatives – 6.4% of 391 male relatives died compared to 3.5% among the 512 female relatives (significant at the $p=0.05$ level). The above information is summarized in tables III and IV.

Some observers, CLAYTON [1974] and PARKERS *et al.* [1969] in particular, have commented on the unusually low mortality rate among the relatives of the controls in this study. The expected death rate is approximately 4.0% in England and Wales while in Llandiloes, where the study was conducted, the death rate was much lower approximately 1%.

COX and FORD [1964] reported results of another prospective study

Table III. Mortality rate of bereaved and nonbereaved relatives for 3 years after index date (expressed as percentages)

	1st year bereaved	non bereaved	2nd year bereaved	non-bereaved	3rd year bereaved	non-bereaved
Spouses	12.2*	1.2*	6.6	3.0	2.5	1.9
Other relatives	3.21**	0.56**	1.99	1.25	n.a.	n.a.

* Significant at the $p=0.01$ level; ** significant at the $p=0.05$ level.
Extrapolated from table V in Rees and Lutkins [1967].

in which they used a different method to ascertain mortality rates of a bereaved population. Using data as to awards of pensions during the year 1933 from the British National Contributory Pension System, they determined that the mortality rate among widowed women was highest during the second 6-month period after bereavement than at any other time during the 5-year follow-up period. During the second 6-month period the ratio of actual to expected death in the widowed was 1–0.08. Cox and Ford report that the mortality rate among the widowed was higher than that of married women although no data was provieded concerning mortality rates of the subjects or the married women. Cox and Ford do acknowledge possible weaknesses in their study. Their finding that the highest mortality rate was during the second 6-month period after bereavement could be an artifact of their methodology; the only information available to them was the date that the widow was awarded the pension. Some time for processing of the widow's claim might have elapsed between their husband's death and the award of the pension and some widows might have died before applying for a pension. Because of limitations in their methods and the limited raw statistical data provided in Cox and Ford's study, it cannot be considered conclusive. However, it is very supportive of the basic hypothesis of increased mortality among the bereaved.

In a more rigorously designed study, Young *et al.* [1963] followed 4,486 widowers, aged 55 years or older, for 5 years after their wives' death. This was the same population that Parkes *et al.* [1969] studied 4 years later. During the first 6 months after bereavement, the mortality rate among the widowers rose 40% as compared to the expected mortality rate among married men of the same age. The Student's t test was performed comparing death rates among both groups and the higher mortality rate among widowers

Table IV. Distribution of relatives who died following bereavement expressed as a percentage of those 'AT RISK' each year

	1st year			2nd year			3rd year			4th year		
	male	female	total	male	female	total	male	female	total	male	female	total
Survey group												
Spouse	19.6	8.5	12.2	4.9	7.1	6.6	7.7	–	2.5	2.8	2.2	2.4
Parent	18.8	10.5	14.3	14.3	–	6.7	9.1	11.6	10.7	–	6.6	3.6
Child	3.0	0.4	1.6	0.5	0.4	0.5	0.5	0.4	0.5	–	–	–
Sibling	4.8	3.9	4.3	0.9	2.7	1.9	0.9	0.7	0.8	2.4	0.7	1.6
Control group												
Spouse	3.9	–	1.2	2.0	3.5	3.0	4.2	0.9	1.9	4.3	–	1.3
Parent	11.0	–	3.4	–	–	–	–	12.5	3.6	–	–	–
Child	–	–	–	1.3	–	0.7	–	–	–	–	–	–
Sibling	0.8	1.4	1.1	1.5	0.7	1.1	–	2.6	1.1	1.6	0.7	1.1

Extrapolated from table V in Rees and Lutkins [1967].

was found to be highly significant statistically (p=0.0001 level). Five years after bereavement, the high mortality rate among the widowers had gradually returned to the same level as the married men.

CLAYTON [1974] reports on the only study that finds no significant increase in the mortality rate among the bereaved. No significant difference in mortality occurred between widowed men and women compared with married men and women matched by age, sex, and geographical location 13 months after bereavement. Only 4% (4 out of 109) of CLAYTON's bereaved sample died during the 1st year of bereavement, compared to a 5% death rate among control subjects (5 out of 109).

Reviewing these studies as a group, we conclude that there is very good evidence to support the hypothesis that the bereaved are greater 'at risk' for overall mortality. With the sole exception of the CLAYTON study all other studies, notably those using large samples, have found a greater mortality rate for the bereaved with trends concerning the greater risks of the relatively young adult bereaved and the finding that the second 6-month period following bereavement is the time of peak risk.

However, certain methodological issues need to be acknowledged. In the retrospective study by KRAUS and LILIENFELD [1959], there might be the fact of 'selection' operating such that widows who remain in good health tend to remarry while those who become ill do not. This would tend to bias both populations so that the sample of widowed would be skewed to the 'unfit' side because more of the healthy widowed might have remarried. The control group of married subjects would also tend to be skewed – to the healthier side. Also, errors in the reporting of census data in terms of misstatements of marital status might be considered as a possible source of data error. Although the YOUNG *et al.* [1963] study was prospective, there was no subject contact and the data came solely from the Registrar General's Office (Great Britain). Error in the study's findings might be present in terms of misinformation in the data obtained through records.

Nevertheless, even with these possible biasing factors, the weight of the evidence supports the hypothesis that the recently bereaved are greater 'at risk' for overall mortality.

Possible Mechanisms Leading to Increased Mortality

Assuming that the evidence presented above in support of the hypothesis is substantiated by further research, the next question that would arise would be to ascertian the possible mechanisms accounting for the higher mortality rate in the bereaved. Some possible mechanisms were outlined by KRAUS and LILIENFELD [1959]. They proposed three hypotheses:

(1) Mutual choice of poor risk mates. Individuals with lower survival potential, knowingly or unknowingly, choose mates with a similar lower survival potential.

(2) Joint exposure to unfavorable environment. Individuals who become widowed have shared and continue to share unfavorable environmental influences which led to the death of the first spouse. These influences might include poor housing, bad nutrition, poor sanitation, high stress, etc.

(3) The effects of widowhood. The event of bereavement and subsequent conditions of widowhood have deleterious effects which result in the excessive death rate. The effects of widowhood would include the impact of grief itself; the new worries and responsibilities of single life; alterations in the diet, work schedule, and recreational life; and reduced income and economic conditions.

YOUNG *et al.* [1963] identified many of the same hypotheses as KRAUS and LILIENFELD and also proposed additional hypotheses to attempt to explain their finding of a 40% rise in the mortality rate among their sample of widowed subjects. Their hypotheses are:

(1) Hogogamy. The tendency for unfit to marry unfit. This is the same hypothesis as proposed by KRAUS and LILIENFELD.

(2) Common infection. This hypothesis is based on CICCIO's [1940] study which found that spouses often die from the same disease.

(3) Joint unfavorable environment. KRAUS and LILIENFELD also proposed this hypothesis.

(4) Loss of care. The widowed have to adapt to a new social role, especially self-care such as nutrition, hygiene, etc., as a result of losing a spouse which may impair their resistance to disease.

(5) Desolation effect. Grief is 'almost certainly' associated with changes in the functioning of the endocrine and central nervous system.

There has been little direct testing of these various hypotheses. The hogogamy hypothesis could easily be tested by determining age at death of couples compared with expected rate of death for same age persons who were not married or by a prospective study of rates of illness in couples. The common infection hypothesis has been disregarded in recent years in modern industrial countries with improved sanitary living conditions, modern health care, and a fall in the death rate from infectious disease. When CICCIO originally proposed this hypothesis in the 1940s, before the advent of antibiotic drugs, there may have been a higher probability of a spouse dying from the same disease because of contagion but it is unlikely nowadays. The joint unfavorable environment hypothesis is probably more plausible than the previous two hypotheses but is as yet undocumented. Of the five hypotheses offered, the final two, the loss of care hypothesis and the desolation effect hypothesis direct attention to the psychobiological effects of grief.

Suicide

Completed Suicides

The previous section reviewed the evidence for a rise in the general mortality among bereaved persons. In this section we examine suicide as one specific cause of death.

McMahon and Pugh [1965] found that the suicide rate among the widowed population was 2.5 times higher in the first 6 months after bereavament and 1.5 times higher during the 1st, 2nd, and 3rd year after bereavement. By 4 years after the loss, the rate had returned to baseline. These figures were based on a study of 320 widowers and widows who had committed suicide in Massachusetts between 1948 and 1952. The suicide sample was compared with a control group matched for age, sex, and race who had died from causes other than suicide. Males were found to have a higher suicide rate than females, among widowed males the age-standardized suicide rate was 3.5 times higher than the suicide rate among married men. Among females, the rate was 2 to 1 comparing the widowed subjects to married controls.

In a striking study, Bunch *et al.* [1971] reported 50% of 75 consecutive suicides in West Sussex, Great Britain had experienced maternal bereavement within 3 years of the suicide. This high maternal bereavement rate in suicides was compared to a 20% maternal bereavement rate among controls who were matched for age, sex, marital status, and geographical location. Moreover, 22% of the suicides, compared to 9% of the controls, had experienced loss of their fathers within the 5 years prior to the suicide. The observed number of maternal deaths among suicides was significantly greater than the expected number of deaths calculated from available life expectancy tables. In addition, marital status of the suicides were also ascertained. Married suicides and controls were not significantly different in respect to loss of a mother, but the single male suicides showed greater recent maternal bereavement (60%) compared to 6% of single male controls. The authors hypothesize that single males may be a 'high risk' group for suicide following their mother's death because of the higher proclivity of males to act out via self-destructive impulses whereas women easily seek out medical and psychiatric help.

KRAUS and LILIENFELD [1959] found similarly high rates for suicide among the males in their retrospective study. The ratio of death by suicide for widowed males as compared to married males was 9.3 to 1 in the 20–24 age group, 6.9 to 1 for ages 24–34, and 3.5 to 1 for men aged 35–44 years. Unfortunately, their study does not report rates for death by suicide for women.

MURPHY and ROBINS [1967] found that in a group of alcoholics who committed suicide 7% (5 out of 31) experienced bereavement of a significant other within 1 year of the suicide. An additional 41% of the alcoholics who committed suicide experienced another type of loss including separation, divorce and other losses. 32% of these other types of loss occurred within 6 weeks of the suicide. MURPHY and ROBINS also found that in a group of suicides who were diagnosed as having an affective disorder after their suicide 5% (3 out of 60) experienced bereavement within 1 year of the suicide. An additional 10% of suicides with affective disorders experienced the other types of losses. The authors concluded that alcoholics were a 'high risk' group for suicide after the loss of an 'affectional relationship'.

Suicide Attempters

LEVI *et al.* [1966] found that 60% of psychiatric inpatients who had attempted suicide had experienced antecedent disruptions of a close interpersonal relationship within 1 year of the attempt. This high rate in the suicide attempters was compared to 50% of patients with suicidal urges and 30% of nonsuicidal psychiatric inpatients. A major weakness of their study is their lack of distinguishing death of a significant other by the relationship to the subject (death of parents, spouse, family are combined). Another finding in the LEVI study is that the suicide attempt group had experienced significantly more childhood separations ($p<0.001$) from significant others before the age of 17 than the other two groups of patients. Although suicide attempt is not suicide death, a trend emerges for the bereaved to be at 'high risk' for suicide and for suicide attempt.

Specific Medical Disorders

The hypothesis that bereavement or 'pathological' grief causes an increase in morbidity and mortality has been studied for several disease systems. These disease systems include: cancer, cardiovascular disease, acute closed angle glaucoma, Cushing's disease, disseminated lupus erythematosus, idiopathic glossodynia, pernicious anemia, pneumonia, rheumatoid arthritis, thyrotoxicosis, tuberculosis, ulcerative colitis, and others. The evidence linking each of these disease systems to bereavement and grief will be discussed in detail in this section.

Cancer

Several investigators have offered evidence that loss of a significant other and the resulting grief increases the incidence of cancer among bereaved persons. Studies have been conducted on the various types of cancer to determine if a relationship exists between bereavement and increased morbidity. Each type of cancer studied will be discussed separately.

Unspecified Neoplasms

LESHAN [1965] reported morbidity rates for unspecified neoplasms. In his sample, 72% of adult cancer patients experienced a significant psychic loss (of a significant person, job, or role change) within 6 months to 9 years prior to onset of the neoplasm, compared to a comparable loss among 10% of healthy controls. A major weakness in LESHAN's retrospective study was that bereavement due to death of a significant other was not distinguished from psychic losses such as job, etc. The lack of a specified time interval between the loss and the onset on the neoplastic disease presents a further methodological problem.

In KRAUS and LILIENFELD's [1959] study, the death rate for malignant neoplasms doubled among the bereaved of all age groups and sexes compared to the death rate due to neoplasms among the married controls.

Cancer of the Breast

BACON *et al.* [1952] reported that 22% (9 out of 40) women with cancer of the breast had experienced a death of a significant other within 2 years of onset of cancer. 50% (20) women reported increasing guilt in the year preceding onset of cancer along with depression, anxiety, self-criticism and self-condemnation.

Contrary to this finding, KRAUS and LILIENFELD [1959] found no significant difference between widows and married women in the death rate due to breast cancer. MUSLIN *et al.* [1965] also found no statistically significant difference with respect to loss of a significant other (a first-degree relative or close friend) between subjects with breast cancer and controls who were in the hospital for a nonmalignant biopsy.

Cancer of the Cervix

This site of cancer has been studied to test the psychodynamic hypothesis that among women external loss would be manifested in female organ changes. KRAUS and LILIENFELD [1959] found a high ratio of cancer of the genital organs in widowed females compared to married controls in their rigorously designed study using a retrospective record search methodology. PALOUCEK and GRAHAM [1965] studied 88 consecutive patients and found that 65% of women with cancer of the ovary, uterine and cervix had experienced a recent 'debilitating' experience. The authors defined a 'debilitating' experience as either a physical illness, such as a respiratory infection; a psychosocial change, such as a death of a husband; or combined physical and psychosocial, such as the patient caring for a mother who had had a stroke. PALOUCEK and GRAHAM did not report the incidence of each type of 'debilitating' experience. Death of a significant other was not discussed separately so its incidence cannot be ascertained. Another methodological weakness of the study was the absence of a control group.

SCHMALE and IKER [1965] using a different methodology than the two studies previously summarized found that among a group of 51 women who came to a hospital for biopsies, psychiatrists forecasted which women would have cancer and which ones would not. The psychiatrists based their judgments on the women's response to an open-ended interview with emphasis on reports of feelings of helplessness or hopelessness during the 6 months prior to the biopsy. The psychiatrists' forecasts were statistically significant (X^2 of 5.29, $p=0.02$ level). They accurately anticipated diagnosis of cancer in 11 cases. The rate of occurrence of death of a loved one was equal among both groups; 1 loss among the 19 women with uterine cancer compared to 1 loss among the 32 women who had nonmalignant bipsies. There was also an equal rate of threat of loss of a loved one among each of the two groups.

SCHMALE and IKER's study was one of the first to separate out the occurrence of actual loss due to death from feelings of helplessness and hopelessness. In the studies previously discussed in this chapter, only the loss by death of a significant other was considered. Most studies take for granted that grief is assumed to automatically follow bereavement. SCHMALE and IKER assessed the psychological state of the patient manifesting a somatic disease to try and determine if the person had grieved according to the criteria of LINDEMANN and ENGEL.

Leukemia and Lymphoma

GREENE [1954, 1956, 1965] has investigated the role of loss and separation among patients with leukemia and lymphoma. In his earliest study (1954) he reported that 85% of men admitted to the hospital with a diagnosis of leukemia and lymphomia (17 out of 20 patients, ages 25–77 years, with an average age of 49 years) had experienced loss or separation from a mother figure, either their wife or mother. Concurrently, the patients were also experiencing psychic losses in other aspects of their lives due to retirement, change of work, injury, etc. No data is reported as to the time interval between incidence of the various types of losses and the onset of leukemia.

In a subsequent study, GREENE *et al.* [1956] reported on 32 women aged 20–71 (average age 42 years) who were admitted to the hospital with diagnosis of leukemia or lymphoma. 75% of these women (24 pateints) had experienced significant losses prior to hospitalization. Among the 12 categories of loss and separation included in this study were: death or threat of death or separation from mother, father, husband, children, or significant others; change or loss of home; loss of work; and menopause. 16 women reported experiencing losses in 3 or more of these 12 categories. 43% (14) of these women experienced death or threat of death or separation from their mothers. Unfortunately, this report does not provide data as to incidence of each category of loss and therefore, loss due to death of a significant other cannot be distinguished from other categories.

In a more rigorously designed retrospecitve study, GREENE [1965] reported that 51% (31 of 61) men age 21–85 (mean age of 58 years) had experienced recent loss or separation from significant others within 4 years of onset of leukemia or lymphoma. 22% (14) had experienced loss of a mother, 8% (5) lost a father, and 20% (12) had lost a wife. Also, 44% (27) men were adjusting to a threatened disability from an anticipated surgical operation, 31% (19) had lost a job, and 34% had recently retired. GREENE hypothesizes that the men developed the onset of the manifest desease in a psychic setting in which they were exposed to loss of personal and emotional support from their mother or a mother figure.

The quality of evidence provided by this set of studies is seriously limited by methodological weakness, especially lack of control groups, small sample size, and problems in ascertainment of types of loss whether actual or psychic. However, there is sufficient evidence to suggest a high incidence of lymphoma and leukemia in recently bereaved persons.

Biological Mechanisms of Cancer

Assuming that these epidemiological trends are substantiated and it is, in fact true, that the bereaved are greater 'at risk' for development of various neoplasms, a number of investigators have speculated as to the possible biological mechanisms which could be operative as intervening processes between bereavement and the growth or dissemination of neoplastic cells. SOLOMON [1969] and SOUTHAM [1969] have attempted to specify possible biological mechanisms by which bereavement and other psychosocial processes might affect the initiation or growth of neoplasms. SOLOMON points out that adrenaline and adrenal corticosteroid output is increased by stress. Various immunologic reactions which recognize and destroy abnormal cells, including possibly cells undergoing neoplastic transformation, are depressed by corticosteroid hormones. Cortisone and desoxycorticosterone also inhibit other defenses such as fibroblastic activity, phagocytosis by neutrophilic leukocytes, and the acute inflammatory reaction to tissue damage.

Moreover, SOUTHAM suggests that smooth muscle activity is altered by adrenaline and autonomic system activity which might influence dissemination of tumor cells, particularly from gastrointestinal neoplasms. SOUTHAM also proposes that, since adrenal corticosteroids and sex steroids affect intravascular clotting mechanisms, the hypercoagulable state, as it results in intravascular depositiaton of fibrin, increases the probability that circulating tumor cells will adhere to and penetrate through capillary walls. SOUTHAM states that each of the mechanisms he identifies is documented so that the sequence is plausible, but it is not yet established as to whether the whole chain of events occurs together.

FREDERICK [1971] also speculates upon the possibility that grief, with the resulting increased corticosteroid levels, might alter immunological-readiness state which might be possibly necessary to fight off the development of the malignancy. Since corticosteroids suppress the immune response, the grieving person might therefore be more susceptible to the malignant transformation of virus than a person who is not experiencing grief or other stress.

It must be acknowledged that these speculations are attempts to identify plausible mechanisms that may link grief to neoplastic growth. These theories rest upon existing research which indicates a relationship between stress response in neuroendocrine systems, particularly the adrenocortical system and pituitary hormones, and vascular and immunological processes known to influence neoplastic growth. It will remain for future research to demonstrate whether or not these possible mechanisms are, in fact, operating in the pathogenesis of neoplasms among recently bereaved individuals. Even if these mechanisms are indeed operating, it is of note that relatively few proponents of the psychosomatic point of view in neoplasm hold that stress or loss, even as direct as bereavement, are a single causative factor. At best, bereavement and grief are considered precipitants activating a neoplastic process in individuals predisposed by genetic, immunological, viral, or other conditions.

Cardiovascular Disease

'Broken heart' is a term commonly used in describing the person who is bereaved. A number of investigators have attempted to test the scientific validity of this folklore relationship. Parkes [1969] attempted to document an increase in mortality due to heart disease among a bereaved population. Parkes' data were from the same sample studied by Young *et al.* [1963] previously mentioned in this chapter. Among the 4,486 widowers aged 55 years and older followed for 9 years, the mortality rate for heart disease in the first 6 months of bereavement was 40% higher than the expected rate for the general population matched for age and sex. The death rate due to coronary thrombosis was 67% higher than that expected for the population and the death rate due to other forms of arteriosclerotic and degenerative heart disease was 60% higher than the expected mortality rate based on national figures for Great Britain for married men of the same age.

Kraus and Lilienfeld [1959] had found similarly high mortality rates for heart disease in a younger bereaved population for both men and women. They found that mortality rates due to arteriosclerotic heart disease and vascular lesions affecting the CNS were 10 times greater among the widowed than among the married controls under age 35. Rates for other froms of heart diseases, such as chronic rheumatic heart disease, nonrheumatic chronic endocarditis and other myocardial degeneration, hypertension with heart disease, and general arteriosclerosis also showed a higher mortality rate among the widowed subjects compared to the rates among the married controls. KRAUS and LILIENFELD concluded that the 'markedly increased risk of dying' from arteriosclerotic heart disease and vascular lesions affecting the central nervous system occurred among the young widowed group.

The evidence from these two studies supports the hypothesis noted since biblical times (Isaiah) that bereavement causes a 'broken heart'. A dramatic instance on the effects of grief is summarized by ENGEL [1971] in his paper 'Sudden and Rapid Death During Psychological Stress'. In a series of 177 instances of rapid death, 44% died during a period of acute grief or while they were in mourning. The time interval between death of a significant other and sudden death of the individual studied was very small, varying from cases of death within minutes to many within weeks or months. The predominant cause of death in the subjects was attributed to cardiovascular causes.

Grief as a special instance of stress may change the blood pressure, heart rate, flow of blood through the coronary arteries, and the clotting ability of the blood. Bereaved people also smoke more. They may also alter their diet in a way to increase coronary thrombosis [PARKES and BROWN, 1972; MADDISON and VIOLA, 1968]. As PARKES and BROWN [1972] speculate, any of these changes could play a part in increasing intravascular clotting within an already diseased coronary artery, thereby precipitaitng coronary thrombosis.

Other Disorders

COHEN and HAJIOFF [1972] studied 52 subjects with *acute closed angle glaucoma.* Of these subjects, 8% experienced bereavement within 8 weeks of onset. In this study subjects were compared to a control group with other visual disorders matched for age, sex, social class, degree of visual impairment and threat to sight. Only 4% of the controls experienced bereavement within the 8 weeks of their onset of disease. This was not a statistically significant difference. When stressful events other than bereavement were assessed (such as surgical operations, moving, separation from significant other, respiratory infections, etc.) a statistically significant difference emerges 38% of the glaucoma subjects compared to 14% of the controls experienced these stressful events within the same time period. Possible mechansims by which grief could produce the acute closed angle glaucoma are described by BOYD and McLEOD [1964] who speculate on the rate that high levels of corticosteroids produced by stress can create alterations in intraocular pressure and can cause induction of glaucoma.

GIFFORD and GUNDERSON [1970] studied 10 patients with *Cushing's disease,* hypercortisolism caused by a disturbance of hypothalamic- pituitary regulation. 80% of the patients, experienced loss through separation or death of a close relationship prior to the onset of symptoms. Among the other 2 patients, one had lost a job with resultant feelings of helplessness and the other had a conflict-ridden marriage. The authors propose that Cushing's disease is a 'psychophysiological response to bereavement or its emotional equivalents, occurring in predisposed individuals with a disturbance in the hypothalamic-pituitary regulation of adrenocortical activity'.

MCCLARY *et al.* [1955] studied 14 patients with *disseminated lupus erythematosus.* They found that 93% of the patients had experienced a 'crisis' in their relationship with significant others during the 4 years prior to onset of the disease. Unfortunately, the authors do not distinguish death of significant others from separations, threat of loss, illness or divorce and there is no data given for any of these types of crises.

HEIMAN [1965] reported on 3 women with *functional uterine bleeding.* In all cases a loss of a significant other occurred, although only one of the losses occurred through death; the other losses were through separation.

SCHOENBERG [1967] reported on *idiopathic glossodynia.* He studied 25 patients who experienced 'burning mouth' and 24% of these patients experienced death or threat of death of a significant other concurrently with onset of symptoms. Findings based on an oral exam and laboratory work-up determined that all of the 8 males and 17 females (average age 54 years) had no physical basis for their complaints.

LEWIN [1959] studied 10 patients with *pernicious anemia.* All of the 8 females and 2 males (average age 50 years) had experienced emotional depression to a marked degree. The patients connected their depression with a recent sudden loss, real or symbolic. These losses included death of a parent, friend; marriage of a child; bankruptcy; and menopause. Deaths of significant others was not distinguished as a separate category. LEWIN hypothesizes that depression may be a factor in the symptomatic state of pernicious anemia by reducing the intrinsic factor (lack of gastric secretion) below the critical level required for normal erythropoiesis. He also suggests that genetic factors cause certain people to be prone to react to stressful life events such as bereavement with pernicious anemia which results from the deficiency of the specific gastric secretion essential for optimal absorption of vitamin B_{12} from the intestines.

KRAUS and LILIENFELD [1959] reported that the death rate among widowed males due to *pneumonia* was 7.7 to 1 in the age 24–34 group compared to the married controls and 6.9 to 1 in the age group of 35–44 years. The ratio was smaller for women.

MEYEROWITZ *et al.* [1968] reported on 8 pairs of female monozygotic twins with *rheumatoid arthritis*. Of the 8 female monozygotic twins with rheumatoid arthritis, 50% (4) experienced psychological stress which the authors term 'entrapment', signifying a situation that the index twin considered enveloping (i.e. from which there was no escape such as the death of a mother leaving care of a psychotic father to the affected twin).

KLEINSCHMIDT *et al.* [1965] studied 84 patients with *thyrotoxicosis* (Grave's disease). 85% of these patients with exophthalamic goiter experienced 'traumatic' events prior to onset of the disease. These traumatic events included death of a significant other, car accident, fantasized attempted rape, and dissolution of a daughter's marriage. No data is given as to the incidence of bereavement as a separate category.

KRAUS and LILIENFELD [1959] found that the mortality rate due to *tuberculosis* among widowed males was increased compared to married males. The rates for females was lower but there was still a higher ratio of tuberculous deaths among widows than among married controls.

Ulcerative colitis has been studied by several investigators concerning a possible relationship to bereavement. LINDEMANN [1945] reported that 58% of this subjects (26 out of 45) had experienced loss of a significant other close to the onset of their ulcerative colitis. An additional 4.5% of subjects had ceased to interact with an 'important person' because of disillusionment or rejection. This 'important person' had a particular significance for the patient manifested by special dependency. LINDEMANN noted that when an ulcerative colitis patient experienced a loss of this significant other, they increased their requests for consultation from the medical service. In a later report, LINDEMANN [1950] described 87 patients with ulcerative colitis of whom 64% (56) had experienced bereavement due to death of significant other. An additional 36% (31) patients experienced other losses such as rejection or disillusionment from the significant other, loss of cultural milieu, or surgical operation. LINDEMANN concluded that 'loss of security, especially the loss of another person of emotional significance, is frequently encountered as the crisis in human relationships which preceded the onset of the illness'.

FELDMAN *et al.* [1967] reported on 34 patients with ulcerative colitis admitted to a gastroenterology unit between August 1964 and June 1966. In their uncontrolled study, 44% (15) of the patients had a 'moderately eventful emotional factor' within 6 months of a relapse. Unfortunately, 'an eventful emotional factor' is not elaborated upon and the study does not say specifically if deaths of significant others is included as an 'emotional factor'.

Illegitimate pregnancy is an interesting area which does not fit into any of the usual disease categories but has a bearing on the effects of bereavement on general health and well-being. GREENBERG *et al.* [1959] reported that 42% of women (13 out of 31) with an out-of-wedlock pregnancy which resulted in a live birth experienced a death of a significant other within a 6-month period prior to conception. Death of a parent occurred in 19% of the women, death of a significant adult in 10%, and death of a fetus during a previous pregnancy occurred in 13%. Other forms of loss through separation occurred in 77% of the women (24 out of 31). These other types of losses included separation from their mother (54%), separation from their father (29%), and separation from other significant adults (17%). The authors hypothesize that a hyperfertile state might occur following loss and mourning.

Patients with other disorders, such as asthma, diabetes mellitus, infectious hepatitis, hypertension, duodenal ulcer, neurodermatitis, and Raynaud's disease, have been discussed in the literature as showing an increase risk during bereavement. However, these reports were too limited to warrant discussion.

Decrease in General Well-Being

In addition to evidence that there is an increase in specific diseases occurring among bereaved persons there is also evidence of a relationship between bereavement and decrease in general well-being.

In discussing the possible decrease in well-being due to bereavement, it is important to distinguish between symptoms which are part of the grief itself from other reactions. ENGEL [1961], LINDEMANN [1945] and CLAYTON [1974] have documented the rapidity with which the grief syndrome appears after the bereavement. Grief usually reaches its peak in the subsequent 4 months of bereavement. By the end of 1 year, 85% of the bereaved are relatively symptom-free. Therefore, studies which describe symptomatology during the first 6 months of bereavement may not be direct tests of an hypothesis of increase in disease susceptibility unless efforts are made to separate out the grief reaction itself.

Symptoms of decrease in well-being are those usually associated with grief. LINDEMANN [1944] described such somatic symptoms as sensations of somatic distress occurring in waves lasting from 20 min to an hour at a time with feelings of tightness in the throat, choking with shortness of breath, need for sighing, an empty feeling in the stomach, lack of muscular power, and an intense subjective distress described as tension or mental pain. ENGEL [1961] also described grief symptoms and behavior in detail.

Several studies have been conducted to determine on a quantitative basis exactly what symptoms a bereaved population experienced. MARRIS [1958] interviewed 72 widows under age 56 years and reported that 43% (31) considered their health to be generally worse since bereavement. The symptoms experienced by the widows included: loss of weight, rheumatism and fibrositis, asthma, bronchitis and cramping pains in the chest, recurrence of duodenal ulcers, gastric ulcers, indigestion, swollen feet and ulcers of the legs, falling hair, skin irritation and rashes, absecesses of the gums, headaches, dizziness and nerves. The widows and their physicians judged that these symptoms were caused or aggravated by their husband's death. No data as to the incidence or severity of the above-mentioned symptoms are given by MARRIS although he mentions that 79% (57) of the widows experienced difficulty sleeping after bereavement.

MADDISON and VIOLA [1968] administered a self-report questionnaire to 375 widows aged 45–60 years, a year after beravement, and to a group of matched controls. New or exacerbated symptoms and complaints reported more frequently by the widows, as compared to the controls, were: trembling, migraine, dizziness, skin rashes, vomiting, weight loss and chest pain.

PARKES and BROWN [1972] administered a questionnaire to 56 widows and widowers and to matched controls asking if the subjects had experienced symptoms during the 13 months since their bereavement. Male widowers reported a significantly greater mean number of acute and autonomic symptoms than their controls. The widowers reported a mean of 2.36 acute symptoms compared to 1.1 acute symptoms among the controls ($t=1.79$, $p<0.05$). Widowers reported a mean of 0.95 autonomic symptoms compared to 0.21 autonomic symptoms among the controls ($t=2.61$, $p<0.02$). There was no significant difference in the mean number of all types of symptoms between the widows and their controls. However, the authors state that seven individual symptoms distinguish between the bereaved subjects and the non-bereaved controls; they are: dizziness or fainting, trembling or twitching, nervousness, chest pains, sweating without cause, lump in the throat, and palpitations. There was a trend for more bereaved to report these symptoms but none of the differences reached statistical significance. Two symptoms did, however, reach statistical significance for the bereaved group; they were: an increase in sleeplessness reported as 'trouble falling asleep' ($p<0.02$) and 'awakening in the middle of the night' ($p<0.001$), and weight fluctuations ($p<0.05$). Both bereaved and nonbereaved women reported a greater number of symptoms than both groups of men to such a degree that the control women reported a larger number of symptoms than the bereaved men. A follow-up study, 2–4 years after bereavement found little difference between symptoms reported by bereaved and nonbereaved men and women.

CLAYTON [1974] reported on 90 widows and widowers (average age 61 years) who were compared with nonbereaved controls matched for age, sex, and geographical location. The only symptoms whose differences in frequency reached statistical significance among the bereaved group during the 1st year of bereavement were: blurred vision (25% of the subjects reported this symptoms compared to 9% of the controls, $p<0.005$) and palpitations (17% of subjects reported this symptom compared to 3% of the controls, $p<0.01$). CLAYTON [personal commun. 1975] also reports that symptoms such as weight loss and sleep distress also attained statistical significance for the bereaved subjects.

MUTTER and SCHLEIFER [1966] studied 42 hospitalized children (ages 6–12 years) and compared them with 45 well children. 67% of the hospitalized children and 46% of the well children had experienced actual or threatened loss of a significant other during the 6-month period prior to admission to the hospital. This difference was statistically significant ($X^2=3.02$, $0.05<p<0.10$). Almost 50% of the ill children had experienced moderate to severely threatening changes in their psychosocial settings (such as serious illness of a family member, departure of a close friend, death of a parent or permanent placement outside of the home, etc.) while none of the well group of children experienced the severely threatening changes and less than 25% experienced moderately threatening changes (such as illness of a family member, departure of a close friend, etc.). The hospitalized children were admitted for acute illness of genitourinary, gastrointestinal, nervous system, respiratory and other systems and not those conventionally considered to be psychosomatic (i.e., ulcerative colitis, asthma, etc.).

In a study on an older age group, STERN *et al.* [1951] studied 25 subjects (aged 53–70 years) at a gerontological unit of the Department of Psychiatry at the University Hospital of McGill in Montreal, Canada. The authors found a dearth of usual psychological manifestations of grief or of conscious guilt feelings, but observed a 'preponderance' of somatic symptoms developing soon after bereavement illustrative of decline in general health. These symptoms included: poor appetite, indigestion, insomnia, anorexia, amnesia, arthritis, breathlessness, accidents, diarrhea, fatigue, and senile dementia. Unfortunately, no data as to incidence of each symptom is reported although six case histories are described in detail.

Only one study did not report a decrease in general well-being among bereaved subjects. HEYMAN and GIANTURCO [1973] reported on 41 elderly subjects aged 60–94 years. The 14 men and 27 women in their sample were evaluated by psychiatric ratings, physical status, and social history. The subjects, who were part of a long-term aging project at Duke University, served as their own controls; having been studied before and after bereavement. There was no significant decrease in general health after widowhood as determined by a physical exam. There were also no differences between men and women in the number of symptoms reported, although the women reported a mild increase in depressive feeling after bereavement. No significant differences in hypochondriasis as measured by the Cavan Adjustment Rating Scale were found. The authors hypothesize that the absence of change in health in the elderly after widowhood is due to the fact that the elderly are psychologically prepared in advance to accept and expect death of their spouse through psychic mechanisms which have generated gradual identification with the role of widowhood before the actual event.

Health-Care Seeking Behavior

Increased Consultations with Physicians

Increased physician consultation and hospitalization is one measure used to determine if there is an increase in morbidity in the bereaved. The rationale behind use of this measure is that bereaved subjects might exaggerate symptomatology in self-reports or interviews as a function of the grief state. There are few studies of self-report of symptoms before and after bereavement so few direct measures of increase in a subject's report of symptoms can be made. Since self-reports form the majortiy of data on morbidity in the bereaved, increased physician visits can provide a better indicator of a true increase in symptoms. The reasoning behind this is: if the person has an increase in symptoms, he/she will be likely to consult a physician.

PARKES is one investigator who uses this method in several studies. In his (1964) study of 44 London widows average age of 60 years, PARKES found that the mean rates of consultation with physician rose from 2.2 consultations per patient per 6-month period during the 18 months prior ot the terminal illness of her husband to a mean of 3.6 consultations during the first 6 months of bereavement. The increase in consultation rates during the first 6 months after bereavement involved 75% (33) of the subjects ($Z = 5.7$, $p < 0.001$). For the over age 65 group, the consultation rate for non-psychiatric symptoms rose from 2.7 consultations per 6-month period during the control time to 7.4 for the first 6 months after bereavement and decreased to 4.3 for the next 6-month period ($p = 0.05$, Wilcoxon test). Vascular and articular affections among the under age 65 group accounted for most of the increase in consultation ($p < 0.05$, Wilcoxon test). This increase in consultations was mainly due to increase in consultations for osteoarthritis ($p = 0.06$, Wilcoxon test).

Maddison and Viola [1968] used a slightly different method than Parkes to ascertain an increase in consultations and hospitalizations in a widowed sample. They studied 378 widows aged 40–60 years (132 in Boston, Mass. and 243 in Sydney, Australia) who reported symptoms on a self-rating scale. These symptom scores were weighted if the subjects had sought medical attention and further weighted if a hospitalization had occurred during the first 13 months of bereavement. There were significant differences between widows and matched controls in reports of several symptoms and complaints.

In a later study, Parkes and Brown [1972] compared the physician consultation and hospitalization rate for a group of 68 widows and widowers under age 45 years and their controls 13 months after widowhood. There was no difference in physician visits or hospitalizations between the bereaved and their controls. 41% (28) of bereaved persons and 43% (29) of controls had consulted a doctor on three or more occasions during the preceding year.

Clayton [1974] also found no significant difference in physician visits or medical and surgical hospitalizations between a group of 90 widows and widowers (average age 61 years) and their controls (matched for age, sex, and geographical location).

Use of Alcohol and Medication

Along with the general decrease in well-being, many of the bereaved subjects in these studies reported a marked increase in their consumption of various pills, alcohol, and tobacco. Parkes [1964] observed that sedative drugs were prescribed 7 times more frequently for widows under the age of 65 years during the first 6 months of bereavement than in the period preceding the bereavement. For widows age 65 and older there was no significant increase in the prescription of sedatives.

In a later study by PARKES and BROWN [1972], 25% (17) of 68 widows under the age of 45 years reported an increase in the consumption of tranquilizers, alcohol, and tobacco during the 13-month period after bereavement. 28% of bereaved subjects reported an increase in smoking as compared to 9% of controls ($p<0.01$ level). Increased consumption of alcohol was reported by 28% of bereaved women compared to 3% of controls ($p<0.01$ level). Initiation of consumption of tranquilizers was reported by 26% of the widows compared to 4% of the controls ($p<0.001$ level). There was no statistically significant difference between bereaved subjects and controls in the consumption of hypnotic drugs.

MADDISON and VIOLA's [1968] study noted a marked increase in sedative and hypnotic drug intake in their sample of 374 widows aged 45–60 years old compared to controls during the 13 months after bereavement. They also noted an increased alcohol consumption among the widows compared to controls ($p=0.001$ level). Tobacco smoking also showed a marked increase ($p=0.001$ level) in the widows.

There was a small but significant difference ($p<0.05$) in the consumption of sleeping pills reported by the 90 widows and widowers (average age 61 years) compared to matched controls in CLAYTON's [1974] study. CLAYTON found no difference in consumption of tranquilizers or other medicine taken for general health between the two groups.

Discussion

We have reviewed the evidence concerning the effects of bereavement on overall mortality, the incidence of specific diseases, and general well-being. Although the evidence is not conclusive, the trends are sufficiently positive to warrant further investigation and to consider the methodological, biological and psychosocial implications of this relationship.

Methodological Issues

Few of the studies reviewed meet all of the criteria for adequate research design and methodology. Most of the studies have employed a retrospective design. Far too many have lacked a concurrent control group. The issue of control is of crucial importance. As was discussed in the introduction of this chapter, baseline figures for the expected rate of loss in a 'normal' population were calculated by IMBODEN *et al.* [1963] who found that about 9% of adult men will experience a death of a significant other within a given year and about 25% will experience some type of loss by separation from a significant other. Although this data provides some general guidelines for evaluating results of specific studies, it cannot be considered sufficiently stable to obviate the need for a concurrent control group in each research design. It is our recommendation that any further research conducted on testing these hypotheses must employ a concurrent control group matched for important demographic characteristics such as age, sex, social class, and marital status.

Furthermore, many of the studies fail to specify the exact types of loss or separation experienced by their subjects and the time interval between these events and the onset of symptoms. Without such information possible causal relationships cannot even be tested, especially hypotheses about psychic loss due to separation, threat of separation, or possible symbolic meanings given by the patient to the vicissitudes of life change. In this paper we have focussed upon actual loss by biological death because of our conviction that this loss represents the 'pure' case and lends itself to the most rigorous analyiss.

The ideal research design would involve a prospective study in which a cohort of persons subjected to loss by bereavement was compared to a concomitant control group. We recognize that this ideal may not always be realizable, and as an approximation, the retrospective construction of such a cohort from vital statistic records or other appropriate sampling techniques is acceptable, although less than ideal

Greater attention also needs to be given to the selection of measures of mortality, morbidity, general health, and health-care seeking behavior. Excessive reliance upon questionnaires and other self-report methods has possible limitations due to response set. Persons who are grieving are likely to have generalized negative and pessimistic response sets and may exaggerate minor complains or increase any tendency to seek health care for complaints or symptoms which they may otherwise cope with by their own resources. Therefore, self-reports and questionnaires need to be supplemented by 'objective' measures, such as scaled tests, clinician reports, etc., which can correct for the possible response set that characterizes the grieving individual.

Possible Biological Mechanisms

As mentioned previously, the weight of evidence is sufficiently strong that a number of investigators have felt justified in speculating upon the possible biological mechanisms which might be activated by grief and which might serve as intervening processes leading to manifest illness.

Much of this speculation has built upon the findings from the general stress research area initiated by SELYE [1959] and continued by endocrinologists and psychophysiologist. This endocrinologic research has identified the neuroendocrinologic role of the hypothalamic-pituitary axis as the central mediator of stress reponses and the adrenal cortex as the major, but not exclusive, peripheral response organ. A relationship between the increased adrenocorticoid activity, blood flow, and homeostasis has been demonstrated by SCHAYER [1967]. The suppression of the inflammatory reponse by steroids and resultant susceptiblity to pathogens has been worked out by FREDERICK [1971]. The importance of the immunologic response has been alluded to earlier in our discussion about neoplastic disease.

Another psychophysiological mechanism whereby stress can influence disease susceptibility involves the increase in proteolytic activity of the plasma with resultant breakdown of fibrotic tissue by the proteolytic enzymes and the impairment of reticuloendothelial system activity. As a result, the response to infection and pathogenic organisms is imparied [BOVARD, 1961].

Psychoendocrine studies by HAMBURG [1973], SACHAR [1972], and MASON [1959] have amply documented the responsivity of the hypothalamic-pituitary system to environmental events in general and psychosocial stress, in particular.

Psychosocial Mechanisms

In addition to biological mechanisms mediating between stress and changes in specific end organs, attention needs to be paid to social- psychological factors. These social-psychological factors are mainly involved in altering the health-care seeking behavior of the bereaved individual. Among the factors implicated have been: type of health service, grief symptoms themselves as a stimulus to consulting a physician, the effect of personal status on reporting of illness, and social and cultural supports. We will amplify upon each of these in turn.

Type of Health Service

It is important to note that approximately half of the studies on health-care seeking behavior were conducted in countries with national health services (PARKES [1964, 1972], MARRIS [1958], REES and LUTKINS [1967], COX and FORD [1964] in Great Britain and MADDISON and VIOLA [1968] in Australia). The other studies were conducted in the United States of America. The availability of free or low cost physician services is one determinant in seeking help. A bereaved person living in a country with national health service or comprehensive insurance would be more inclined to visit a physician if access was easier and cost reduced. Unfortunately, no studies have been done on health care utilization in the United States by a bereaved population controlling for economic factors such as health insurance coverage or income.

Grief Itself as a Stimulus to Consulting a Physician

The symptoms and distress of grief itself can serve as an important stimulus to consulting a physician. Increased health-care seeking behavior, such as consulting a physician or ingestion of tranquilizers or of other medications, are often responses to the specific symptoms of grief and the attendant temporary impairment of the bereaved individual's usual coping capacity. This response is usually heightened if the deceased has been a strong figure in the bereaved individual's life and one upon whom he/she has depended. The act of seeking medical attention serves not only to relieve specific distressing symptoms but also provides support, reassurance, and nurturance. STOECKLE *et al.* [1964] have documented the importance of psychological distress, especially when experienced as a depressed emotion, in the decision to consult a physician.

Effect of Personal Status on Reporting of Illness

Health-care seeking behavior is influenced by many factors. In addition to symptomatic distress, the availability of health insurance and other economic factors, and social and cultural supports, the patient's response set and attitudes are powerful influences. A number of students of psychosomatic medicine such as HINKLE and CHRISTENSON [1958], PARKES and BROWN [1972] and PARKES [1970] have stated that the meanings that patients give to their symptoms may be more crucial than the actual life situation. Specifically, a person's perceptions of their symptoms as serious or threatening has more to do with their psychological state at the time than the actual 'seriousness' of their symptoms from a medical point of view [MECHANIC, 1964].

Social and Cultural Supports

The extent to which the bereaved individual may utilize the health care system must be seen in relationship to the patient's other available familial, social, and cultural supports. There are major cultural group differences in the availability and types of supporting social networks which assist the bereaved. With the decline of the neighborhood, the extended family, and religious institutions; the traditional social support systems in western society; the bereaved are more likely to seek health care especially from a physician. Widows and other bereaved who do not have access to extended family or who are separated geographically from members of their family would, therefore, be more likely to visit a physician. ZOLA [1966] has pointed to the importance of ethnic and cultural group differences with respect to pain and reasons for seeking assistance for ailments. It would seem reasonable to extend such an approach to cultural differences and ethnic group responses to bereavement but this has not yet been done beyond the anecdotal level. MARRIS [1958] reports that the difference between widows who recovered from their grief in a shorter time and those who took longer to recover was a feeling of support from their relatives. Those widows who felt that they did not get emotional support from their relatives took a longer time to recover and experienced more serious grief reactions.

Conclusions

The research evidence presented in this paper indicates that persons experiencing bereavement are 'greater at risk' for mortality, increased morbidity due to specific disease, decrease in general well-being, and will seek health-care with greater frequency. The epidemiologic research indicates that among the bereaved, the group most 'at risk' are young men under age 45 years, who have lost their wife or mother. With increasing age, the impact of bereavement seems to lessen, but these trends remain to be substantiated by further research.

Clearly the impact of bereavement and resultant grief upon physical health and general well-being has important clinical, epidemiologic, and research implications. Clinically, the clinicians can obviously benefit from epidemiologic research which identifies 'high risk' groups. Research on the specification of various physiological and psychosocial mechanisms can render health planning more effective for both the individual and the group. Hopefully, this will lead to preventive measures which can alleviate the current high rates of mortality, morbidity, and the stress associated with grief.

Bereavement and resultant grief provide an unusual 'experiment of nature'. As such they are the limiting case of the stress and loss hypotheses so widely discussed in current thinking in psychosomatics and psychophysiology. Careful investigation of the bereaved, whether they grieve or not, therefore allows a quasi-experimental approach to testing the impact of important biological phenomenon such as adaptation, stress, loss, attachment bonding and its disruption, and the importance of affiliations in the maintenance of homesostasis and health. As such, further knowledge of this area can contribute immensely to any general theory of health and illness.

Bereavement represents one specific form of stress. Extensive research into psychobiological mechanisms of adaptation to stress has focussed on the neurophysiological, endocrine, and autonomic nervous system mechanisms as an important component of the repertoire of human coping responses. These capabilities are a result of an extensive evolutionary process which humans share with primates and other mammals.

The grief response highlights one aspect of human evolution which has further augmented the adaptive response to stress. Whereas all mammals have evolved affiliative bonding, particularly between mother and infant, for primates in general and humans in particular these bonds are intense, prevasive, and enduring. Given the prolonged period of extrauterine development of primates and humans, the helplessness of the infant renders biologically important the attachment bonding to insure that nurturing and care of the infant takes place to support their biological survival. Thus, bonding between infant and adult and between siblings has great biological adaptive significance for the species and for the individual [HAMBURG, 1973; KLERMAN, 1974].

Disruption of this bond, by loss or separation, almost always initiates profound and intense psychobiological, affective, and psychosocial responses on the part of the individual and the group. Grief is the prototype of this response to the disruption of attachment bonds. Although we do not know the exact neurophysiologic and neurochemical mechanisms which perpetuate these bonds, they probably employ the reward and reinforcement systems located in the subcortical centers closely interactive with hypothalamic, limbic, and other centers regulating neuroendocrine, sympathetic, and arousal functions.

As HAMBURG [personal commun., 1974] and others have pointed out, during most of human history the individual has been involved continually in his/her primary familial group. Given the high infant mortality rate, high death rate from infections, and generally low life expectancy until the recent centuries, the wonder is that the intense distressing nature of grief has not been more maladaptive and disruptive for the individual, the group, and the species. It may well be that the presence of traditional powerful group bonds, such as the extended family and the proximate neighborhood group, has served as important buffers mitigating against the disruptive influence of grief. In recent centuries, however, with increased geographic mobility and the value placed upon independence many adults have voluntarily separated themselves from their primary families. This separation causes the traditional group supports to become less available to modern mankind for coping with loss and grief. Thus, though our mechanisms for handling stress in general and grief in particular have had a long evolutionary development, group and social supports have until very recently been predicated upon stable, enduring, and affiliative relationships which have fostered group membership. The emphasis our society places nowadays on values of independence and autonomy act in a negative way on stable relationships and resulting group supports. It may well be that one of the prices we have paid for modernity is an increased vulnerability to grief.

Seen in this light, the current interest in grief and loss responds to the awareness that the traditional buffering social mechanisms, such as the extended family, the neighborhood, and religious institutions are no longer utilized or valued. In the absence of alternatives, the health and medical care institutions are called upon for nurturance, support, and guidance as well as the relief of specific symptoms by modern technical medical science.

References

Alexander, F.: Emotional factors in essential hypertension. Psychosom. Med. *1:* 173 (1939).

Bacon, C.L.; Renneker, R., and Cutler, M.: A psychosomatic survey of cancer of the breast. Psychosom. Med. *14:* 453–460 (1952).

Bovard, E.W.: A concept of hypothalmus functioning. Perspect. Biol. Med. *5:* 52–60 (1961).

Boyd, T.A.S. and McLeod, L.E.: Circadian rhythms of plasma corticoid levels. Ann. N.Y. Acad. Sci. *117:* 597–613 (1964).

Bunch, J.; Barraclough, B.; Nelson, B., and Sainsbury, P.: Suicide following death of parents. Social Psych. *6:* 193–199 (1971).

Ciccio, A.: On mortality in husbands and wives. Hum. Biol. *12:* 508 (1940).

Clayton, P.: Mortality and morbidity in the first year of widowhood. Archs. gen. Psychiat. *125:* 747–750 (1974).

CLAYTON, P.; DESMARIS, L., and WINOKUR, G.: A study of normal bereavement. Am. J. Psychiat. *125:* 64–74 (1968).

COBB, S. and LINDEMANN, E.: Cocanut Grove burns: a neuropsychiatric observation. Ann. Surg. *117:* 814–824 (1943).

COHEN, S.I. and HAJIOFF, J.: Life events and the onset of acute closed-angle glaucoma. J. psychosom. Res. *16:* 335-341 (1972).

COX, P.R. and FORD, J.R.: The mortality of widows shortly after widowhood. Lancet *i:* 163–164 (1964).

ENGEL, G.: Is grief a disease. Psychosom. Med. *23:* 18–23 (1961).

ENGEL, G.: The psychological setting of somatic disease. The 'giving-up – given-up complex'. Proc. R. Soc. Med. *60:* 553 (1967).

ENGEL, G.: Sudden and rapid death during psychological stress. Ann. intern. Med. *74:* 771–782 (1971).

FELDMAN, F.; CANTOR, D.; SOLL, S., and BACHRACH, W.: Psychiatric study of a consecutive series of 34 patients with ulcerative colitis. Br. med. J. *iii:* 14–17 (1967).

FREDERICK, J.F.: Physiological reactions induced by grief. Omega *2:* 71–75 (1971).

FREUD, S.: Mourning and melancholia (1917); in complete works of Sigmund Freud, vol. 4 (Hogarth, London 1956).

GIFFORD, S. and GUNDERSON, J.G.: Cushing's disease as a psychosomatic disorder. A review of the literature. Perspect. Biol. Med. *13:* 169–221 (1970).

GOODALL-VAN LAWICK, J.: Paper presented at the American Psychosomatic Society, Philadelphia 1974.

GRANT, I.; KYLE, G.C.; TEICHMAN, A., and MENDELS, J.: Recent life events and diabetes in adults. Psychosom. Med. *36:* 121–128 (1974).

GREENBERG, N.H.; LOESCH, J.G., and LAKEN, M.: Life situations associated with the onset of pregnancy. I. The role of separation in a group of unmarried pregnant women. Psychosom. Med. *21:* 296–311 (1959).

GREENE, W.: Psychological factors and reticuloendothelial disease. I. Observations on a group of men with lymphomas and leukemias. Psychosom. Med. *16:* 220 (1954).

GREENE, W.: The psychological setting of the development of leukemia and lymphoma. Ann. N.Y. Acad. Sci. *125:* 794–801 (1965).

GREENE, W.; YOUNG, L., and SWISHER, S.: Psychological factors and reticuloendothelial disease. II. Observations on a group of women with lyphomas and leukemias. Psychosom. Med. *18:* 284 (1956).

HAMBURG, D.: Emotions in the perspective of human evolution; in KNAPP Expression of the emotions of man (Intl. Univ. Press, New York 1973).

HARLOW, H.F.; HARLOW, M.K., and SUOMI, S.J.: From thought to therapy: lessons from a primate laboratory. Am. Scient. *59.* 538–549 (1971).

HEIMAN, M.: The role of stress situations and psychological factors in functional uterine bleeding. J. Mt Sinai Hosp. *23:* 154 (1965).

HEYMAN, D.K. and GIANTURCO, D.T.: Long-term adaptation by the elderly to bereavement. J. Geront. *28:* 359–362 (1973).

HINKLE, L.E. and CHRISTENSON, W.: An investigation of the relation between life experience, personality characteristics, and general susceptibility to illness. Psychosom. Med. *1958:* 278.

HOLMES, T.H. and RAHE, R.H.: The social readjustment rating scale. J. psychosom. Res. *11:* 213–218 (1967).

HUDGENS, R.W.; MORRISON, J.R., and BARCHKA, R.G.: Life events and onset of primary affective disorders. A study of 40 hospitalized patients and 40 controls. Archs. gen. Psychiat. *16:* 134–145 (1967).

IMBODEN, J.B.; CANTER, A., and CLUFF, L.: Separation experiences and health records in a group of normal adults. Psychosom. Med. *25:* 433 (1963).

KASL, S.V. and COBB, S.: Some psychological factors associated with illness behaviors and selected illnesses. J. chron. Dis. *17:* 325 (1964).

KLEINSCHMIDT, H.J.; WAXENBERG, S.F., and CUKER, R.: Psychophysiology and psychiatric management of thyrotoxicosis. A two years follow-up study. J. Mt Sinai Hosp. *23:* 131 (1965).

KLERMAN G.L.: Depression and adaptation: in FRIEDMAN and KATZ The psychology of depression (Winston-Wiley, Washington 1974).

KRAUS, A.S. and LILIENFELD, A.M.: Some epidemiological aspects of the high mortality rate in the young widowed group. J. chron. Dis. *10:* 207–217 (1959).

LESHAN, L. and WORTHINGTON, R.E.: Loss of cathexes as a common psychodynamic characteristic of cancer patients. An attempt at statistical validation of a clinical hypothesis. Psychol. Rep. *2:* 183–193 (1958).

LEVI, L.; FALES, C.H.; STEIN, M., and SHARP, V.H.: Separation and attempted suicide. Archs. gen. Psychiat. *15:* 158–164 (1966).

LEWIN, K.K.: The role of depression in the production of illness in pernicious anemia. Psychosom. Med. *21:* 23–26 (1959).

LINDEMANN, E.: The symptomatology and management of acute grief. Am. J. Psychiat. *101:* 141 (1944).

LINDEMANN, E.: Psychiatric factors in the treatment of ulcerative colitis. Archs. Neurol. Psychiat. *53:* 322 (1945).

MADDISON, D.C., and VIOLA, A.: The health of widows in the year following bereavement. J. psychosom. Res. *12:* 297–306 (1968).

MARRIS, P.: Widows and their families (Routledge & Kegan, London 1958).

MASON, J.W.: Psychological influences on the pituitary and adrenal cortical system: in Recent progress in hormone research (Academic Press, New York 1959).

MCCLARY, A.; MEYER, E., and WEITZMAN, E.: Observations on the role of the mechanism of depression in some patients with disseminated lupus erythematosus. Psychosom. Med. *17:* 310–320 (1955).

MCMAHON, B. and PUGH, T.F.: Suicide in the widowed. Am. J. Epidem. *81:* 23–31 (1965).

MECHANIC, D. and VOLKART, H.: Stress, illness behavior, and the sick role. Am. sociol. Rev. *26:* 51 (1961).

MEYER, A.: in LIEF The commonsense psychiatry of Dr. Adolf Meyer (McGraw-Hill, New York 1948).

MEYEROWITZ, M.; JACOX, R., and HESS, D.W.: Monozygotic twins discordant for rheumatoid arthritis. A genetic, clinical, and psychological study of 8 sets. Arthritis Rheum. *11:* 1–21 (1968).

MURPHY, G.E.: 'Life stress' in a normal population. A study of 101 women hospitalized for normal delivery. J. nerv. ment. Dis. *134:* 150–161 (1962).

MUSLIN, H.; KALMAN, G., and PEIPER, W.J.: Separation experience and cancer of the breast. Ann. N.Y. Acad. Sci. *125:* 802–806 (1965).

MUTTER, A.Z. and SCHLEIFER, M.J.: The role of psychological and social factors in the onset of somatic illness in children. Psychosom. Med. *28:* 333–343 (1966).

MYERS, J.K.; LINDENTHAL, J.J., and PEPPER, M.: Life events and psychiatric impairment. J. nerv. ment. Dis. *152:* 149–157 (1971).

PALOUCEK, F.P. and GRAHAM. J.B.: The influence of psychosocial factors on the prognosis on cancer of the cervix. Ann. N.Y. Acad. Sci. *125:* 814–819 (1965).

PARKES, C.M.: Recent bereavement as a cause of mental illness. Br. J. Psychiat. *110:* 198 (1964a).

PARKES, C.M.: Effects of bereavement on physical and mental health. A study of the medical records of widows. Br. med. J. *ii:* 274–279 (1964b).

PARKES, C.M.: The first year of bereavement. A longitudinal study of the reaction of London widows to the death of their husbands. Psychiatry *33:* 444–467 (1970).

PARKES, C.M.; BENJAMIN, B., and FITZGERALD, R.G.: Broken hearts: a statistical study of increased mortality among widowers. Br. med. J. *i:* 740 (1969).

PARKES, C.M. and BROWN, R.: Health after bereavement. A controlled study of young Boston widows and widowers. Psychosom. Med. *34:* 449–461 (1972).

PAYKEL, E.S.; MYERS, J.K.; DIENELT, M.N., and KLERMAN, G.L.: Life events and depression. A controlled study. Archs. gen. Psychiat. *21:* 753 (1969).

RAHE, R.H. and ARTHUR, R.J.: Life events surrounding illness onset. J. psychosom. Res. *11:* 341–345 (1968).

RAHE, R.H.; MEYER, M.; SMITH, M.; KJAER, G., and HOLMES, T.H.: Social stress and illness onset. J. psychosom. Res. *8:* 35–44 (1964).

REES, W. and LUTKINS, S.G.: Mortality of bereavement. Br. med. J. *iv:* 13–16 (1967).

SACHAR, E.J.; BERGSMAN, A.; MCDONALD, R.K., *et al.:* Corticosteroid response to psychotherapy of depression. I. Evaluations during confrontation of loss. Archs. gen. Psychiat. *16:* 461 (1967).

SCHMALE, A.: Relationship of separation and depression in disease. A report on a hospitalized medical population. Psychosom. Med. *20:* 259–277 (1958).

SCHMALE, A. and IKER, H.: The psychological setting of uterine cervical cancer. Ann. N.Y. Acad. Sci. *125:* 794–801 (1965).

SCHOENBERG, B.: Psychogenic aspects of the burning mouth. N.Y. St. dental J. *33:* 467 (1967).

SCHOENBERG, B.; CARR, A.C., and KUTSCHER, A.H.: The burning mouth syndrome. N.Y. St. J. Med. *71:* 1832–1837 (1971).

SCOTT, J.P. and SENAY, E.C.: Separation and depression: clinical and research aspects (AAAS, Washington 1973).

SELYE, H.: Perspectives in stress research; in Perspectives in biology and medicine, vol. II/4 (Univ. Chicago Press, Chicago 1959).

SETHI, B.B.: Relationship of separation to depression. Archs. gen. Psychiat. *10:* 486–495 (1964).

SOLOMON, G.F.: Emotions, stress, the central nervous system and immunity. Ann. N.Y. Acad. Sci. *164:* 335–343 (1969).

SOUTHAM, C.: Emotions, immunology, and cancer: How might the psyche influence neoplasia? Ann. N.Y. Acad. Sci. *164:* 473–475 (1969).

STERN, K.; WILLIAMS, G.M., and PRADOS, M.: Grief reactions in later life. Am. J. Psychiat. *58:* 289–294 (1951).

STOECKLE, J.D.; ZOLA, I.K., and DAVIDSON, G.E.: The quantity and significance of psychological distress in medical patients. Some preliminary observations about the decision to seek medical aid. J. chron. Dis. *17:* 959 (1964).

WOLFF, H.G.: in WOLF and GOODELL Stress and disease (Thomas, Springfield 1953).

YOUNG, M.; BERNARD, B., and WALLIS, G.: The mortality of widowers. Lancet *ii:* 454–456 (1963).

ZOLA, I.K.: Culture and symptoms. An analysis of patients' presenting complaints. Am. Soc. Rev. *31:* 615–630 (1966).

G.L. KLERMAN, MD, Professor of Psychiatry, Harvard Medical School, Massachusetts General Hospital, *Boston, MA 02114* (USA)

J.E. IZEN, B.A., Research Analyst, Massachusetts General Hospital, *Boston, MA 02114* (USA)

Adv. psychosom. Med., vol. 9, pp. 105–131 (Karger, Basel 1977)

Migration and Physical Illness

IAN PRIOR

Epidemiology Unit, Wellington Hospital, Wellington

Contents

'It is changes that are chiefly responsible for disease, especially the violent alterations.'
HIPPOCRATES

Introduction

Migration is a most important and worldwide phenomenon, and yet the way in which this may influence the health of the migrant and his family has not been thoroughly studied. Doubt still remains as to whether the process results in improvements or a deterioration of the health of the migrant and examples are available in the literature recording changes in each of these directions.

These results are not surprising since the process can represent such a range of changes in environment and of living patterns. There is a need for better standardisation of the type and pattern of migration so that more effective comparisons can be made between studies in different parts of the world. The development of epidemiology as a research discipline applying its methods to 'things that happen to people' is well described by one of the leaders of British epidemiology, J.N. MORRIS [1], in his 1972 Presidential address to the Section of Epidemiology and Prevention of the Royal Society of Medicine. This states clearly the sort of contribution we can expect from epidemiology in the future if it is properly applied. The study of migration in this way, with properly defined samples and criteria is in fact a recent development and this explains the relative lack of medical literature. It is now being realised that well planned and implemented studies of migrant populations have an important contribution to make in extending knowledge concerning such disorders as hypertension, coronary heart disease, bronchitis asthma, mental ill health, suicide, individual and family disorganisation.

The present contribution will review briefly some of the major migrations that are occurring, that have been, or could be available for study. The report will then concentrate on some of the findings that are coming forward from migrant studies relating to blood pressure patterns and hypertension, coronary heart disease, bronchitis and asthma. These disorders constitute major causes of morbidity and mortality in developed countries and are now becoming more important in the developing ones where large numbers of subjects are involved in migration from traditional rural areas to crowded urban industrial centres.

Some examples will be chosen from the area of the Pacific because this forms the area of major research involvement of the author and the group he is associated with.

Migration Patterns

Wherever one looks in the world today there is evidence of people on the move. The motivation is usually to seek, but not always find, improved material resources as an individual or as part of a family; to take part in the greater opportunities for involvement in the 'advantages' of the developed societies; and in many cases to move to an area where educational opportunities will be greater both for the individual, but more commonly for the families of the migrants. At the same time many major migrations such as the movement from Southern to Central Western Europe are looked on as temporary with the aim of returning 'home' when sufficient money has been earned.

Within the Pacific – temporary migrations from the Kingdom of Tonga and from Fiji to Australia and New Zealand come into this same category and carry with them their own particular hazards to physical and mental health.

There is also within the Pacific area more permanent migration occurring from the atolls and high islands of the Cook Islands, Western Samoa, Niue and the Tokelau Islands to New Zealand so that the total number of Pacific Islanders in New Zealand has increased from around 1,900 in 1946 just after the Second World War to around 50,000 in 1973.

Migration and urbanisation are very closely linked in that almost all migration involves the migrant moving into a town or city that contrasts very strongly with his place of departure. The migration of some of the Jewish groups from Northern Africa to Israel, West Indians to the cities of Great Britain, rural blacks from the Southern States to the Northern cities such as New York, Detroit and Chicago are in this category. The movement of people within the Arab countries of the Middle East and Northern Africa in the developing African states can also be mentioned as areas now offering opportunities for study of the problems of migrants.

Within New Zealand, the Maori people have been involved in very major rural/urban migration so that the percentage of their population living in towns or cities has increased from around 15% in 1946 to 70% in 1973. The total population in New Zealand is 3 million of whom 270,000 are classed as Maori – being half caste or more. Considerable intermarriage has occurred since the Europeans came to the country and the number of people with some Maori blood but classed as Europeans is large. The bicultural nature of the society, the emphasis on social and family factors contributing to the functioning of the extended family group of the Maori compared with the nuclear family of the European white New Zealander, and the way which these factors are influenced by the major rural to urban migration offer most valuable opportunities for study of the health and social problems resulting from migration.

A special place must be preserved for those groups involved in 'forced migrations' where the controlling governments have for particular reasons insisted on whole populations being moved. The forced migration of the inhabitants of the tiny rocky island of Tristan da Cunha will be chosen as the example of this type which had for the most part disastrous effects on their health so that when given the opportunity, the majority returned to their barren island and subsistence economy [2].

Classification of Migration

RAVENSTEIN [3] in 1885 first formulated his 'migration laws' and since that time a substantial literature has appeared concerned with the spatial mobility of populations. The UN has produced valuable leads in defining various concepts used in population studies [4, 5].

The term mobility is used to describe all kinds of territorial movements, both temporary and permanent over various distances. An operational definition of migration requires that both temporal and locational criteria are more specifically defined.

If there is interest in the direction of the move, and there almost always is, the distinction is made between in-migrants and out-migrants when describing internal migrations within the one country while for external migrations the terms immigrant and emigrant are used. Migration takes place from an area of origin (departure) to one of destination (arrival) and a group of migrants with a common origin and destination is called a migration stream. Usually, each stream has a counter-stream; the distinction between the two is based on the size of the respective flows. The term gross migration refers to the total number of in-migrants and out-migrants of an area and is sometimes referred to as the turnover of an area. The differences between the two streams would be net migration or balance of migration which may be positive or negative for an area.

Geographical or spatial mobility includes all sorts of moves both temporary and permanent. Social moblity refers to a change in socioeconomic status. Increasingly however, these two types of mobility are treated jointly and measures of these are introduced into migration studies. To explain the mechanism of migration it is necessary to consider the decision-making process and this is best thought of in terms of the 'push and pull' concept. When persons, with a permanent residence decide that their needs can no longer be adequately satisfied at that place and that a move somewhere else is to be considered then a 'push' factor appears. Real life examples include loss of employment, inadequate opportunities, racial, religious or political persecution, social cultural or personal alienation from the community, social or natural disaster. On the other hand, an individual can be satisfied with the present situation but new information may persuade that a move elsewhere will provide new and attractive opportunities including better political, economic, social and material opportunities and these can be termed as 'pull' factors. These ideas are well reviewed in the introduction to a publication *Studies on Internal Migration* [6], where the editors KOSINSKI and PROTHERO stress the way in which numerous positive and negative factors are considered by the migrant in deciding whether to move and where to go. They also stress that decisions may be modified by real or perceived obstacles which include costs and fatigue of move, personal anxiety which will result from the change in the social and physical environment and also the legal restrictions that may need to be dealt with.

MABOGUNJE [7] conceptualises this problem more as a circular interdependent, progressively complex and self-modifying system in which the effects of changes in one part can be traced through the whole system. The migration system is influenced by an economic, social, political and technological environment with an open and continuous interchange between this environment and the migration system. This system approach appears to have considerable merit and the factors that contribute to health and disease can be readily considered within this system. Having received the stimulus, the potential migrant will be influenced by the rural control subsystem (family, local community) in the decision either to remain in the area or make a move. The urban control system (mostly related to family already there, housing and economic opportunity) can help the migrant to adjust to the new environment and eventually become completely settled in the urban setting. Success or failure is constantly transmitting positive or negative feedback to the areas of origin to influence subsequent migration. This certainly serves as a useful model for the migration that is occurring from the South Pacific Polynesian territories to New Zealand, of which the Tokelau Island migration is an example [8].

Research Orientations and Conceptual Framework of Migrant Studies

The question of migration and physical illness is very dependent on the major scientific questions that must be asked in any multidisciplinary study of the process whether the emphasis is on health and disease, geographical or other factors.

Who migrates? What are their particular characteristics? Are they different from nonmigrants?
Why do they migrate?
What are the patterns of flow and direction of the movement and what factors are influencing these?
What are the consequences of migration? What effect does it have on the society of origin, at destination and on the migrants themselves? The consequences can be observed and measured in economic, social, cultural, health, political and demographic terms providing the studies are set up with sufficient skill and resources of personnel and funds to carry them through for the time required to document the changes that occur. The establishment of such multidisciplinary studies has received considerable encouragement and direction through different aspects of the International Biological Program and the Man and the Biosphere Programme.

The methods of contemporary epidemiological research form a key part of such investigations but results will be dependent on the quality and originality of the questions being asked. These relate particularly to the process of adaptation of the migrant in his new setting, the mechanisms involved, the strategies adapted and how these influence overall health and risk to health.

The strategy of migrant studies has been considerably influenced by the concepts of SELYE [9] and the 'general adaptation syndrome', with emphasis on how the hypothalamus pituitary adrenal axis play a part in dealing with a variety of 'stressful' situations both physical and psychosocial. DUBOS [10] from his experience of microbial disease has pointed out how the emergence of microbial disease is not necessarily due to exposure to a new micro-organism, but in a large number of cases is due to factors which disturb the balance between the existing ubiquitous organisms and the host that is harbouring them. The process of migration and urbanisation is often associated with physical crowding at the destination point, but DUBOS' contribution suggests that other environmental factors may affect the homeostatic mechanisms of the host which profoundly influences his susceptibility to disease. Evidence is now accumulating that *it is the presence of other members of the same species* and the relationships between them that could be of key importance in the diseases that emerge following migration and urbanisation.

This concept of the human factor, the effect of man upon man has been developed further by the innovative and original contributions of such workers in the field as CASSEL [11], SYME [12], CHRISTENSON and HINKLE [13], and RAHE [14]. They have contributed towards clearer ideas on the ways in which changes associated with migration, urbanisation and life changes may influence health and disease. Their ideas have provided the basis of hypotheses that can and are being tested in migrant studies.

The theme linking the thinking of these different workers relates to the way in which 'stress' variously defined, results in an overall increased predisposition to disease, both morbidity and mortality, and that it is the interaction of man with his fellows and the ways in which he has been prepared to deal with new situations in his interaction with people and his environment that will influence the outcomes. The presence of 'stressors' and 'protectors', the latter limiting and protecting the individual from noxious agents needs to be emphasized.

The physiological mechanisms involved operate through the hypothalamus, pituitary adrenal cortex axis, and the ability to measure hormone outputs, particularly catecholamines, have added strength to the theoretical basis of these concepts.

The fact that psychosocial factors involved in the process of migration and in the adaptation to this change are of importance is the justification for setting out in the next section some of the hypotheses being considered in this field. They form a suitable basis from which certain specific physical disorders or illnesses will be considered. This does not make the assumption that physical illnesses can readily be considered separate from the psychosocial factors that contribute to them and may also be a part of the individuals response to their presence.

It is also most important to recognise that the migrant is in many cases involved in environmental changes which may contribute to higher risk for certain diseases, particular when they move from a 'low risk' to a 'high risk' environment. Examples include diet, saturated fat, salt use and fibre content, availability of alcohol and tobacco that may contribute to cardiovascular risk, and this forms the second major hypothesis that needs to be tested in prospective migrant studies.

Hypotheses

CASSEL [11, 20] in his various writings has put forward three major hypotheses that appear highly relevant and require testing in migration and urbanisation studies. These have received some input from a variety of animal studies [15] as well as from human studies.

(1) In human populations, when for various reasons, individuals do not receive any feedback or evidence that their actions are leading to desirable

or anticipated consequences, increased susceptibility to disease should occur. In particular this would be true when these actions should allow the individual to modify his relationship to the important social group with whom he interacts. Migrants, in a new situation, unfamiliar with the moves and expectations of the society in which they now live may find that their actions are unlikely to lead to the consequences they anticipate and thus through the physiological mechanisms mentioned above, become more susceptible to disease than those for whom the situation is familiar. SCOTCH [16] and his work among Zulus provides some circumstantial evidence for this. He found that blood pressure levels among the Zulu who had recently migrated to a large urban centre were higher than those in their rural urban setting and also higher than those who had lived for over 10 years in the city.

Cross-sectional studies of this nature are vulnerable, however, since the initial characteristics of the migrants were not measured and it could be argued that they may have had higher blood pressures prior to migration. This emphasises the need for longitudinal studies with definition of the characteristics of the migrant prior to migration. Such studies must document not only the psychosocial cultural factors but also changes in environmental variables including diet and life style patterns.

In two independent studies SYME *et al.* [17, 18] have shown that occupationally and residentially mobile people have a higher prevalence of coronary heart disease than stable populations, and that those individuals displaying the greatest discontinuity between childhood and adult situations as measured by occupation and place of residence have higher rates than those in which less discontinuity could be determined.

STAMLER *et al.* [19] found that the blood pressure and rates of significant hypertension in black migrants to Chicago with less than 10 years in the city were lower than those born in Chicago, those with 10–15 years in Chicago were equal while those with more than 15 years in Chicago were higher than the Chicago born. In fact, these findings could relate to the long-term effect of environmental variables rather than to social stress effects.

(2) The second major hypothesis put forward from the animal work reviewed by CASSEL [11, 20] is that not all members of a population are equally susceptible to the effects of these social pressures. The animal work examining blood pressure and other variables has shown that the more dominant animals show the least effects while the subordinate ones demonstrate the more extreme responses.

The higher levels of blood pressure and hypertensive disease in the blacks in the US compared with the whites could be cited as an example of a group who are often in the subordinate position and who are at particular risk from social and family disorganisation. The National Health Survey conducted by the United States Public Health Service in 1960–1962 showed the prevalence of abnormally elevated blood pressure in urban blacks was 21.1% compared to 13.5% for urban whites. Since that time mortality rates have shown a decline for hypertensive disease that is less in the black than in the white.

(3) A third principle put forward by CASSEL is concerned with the available protective factors which 'buffer' or 'cushions' the individual from the physiological or psychological consequences of these social processes. These protective factors will be biological and social. The biological category would include the adaptive capacities of all living organisms, the capacity, given time, to adjust physiologically and psychologically to a variety of environmental circumstances. This is a human characteristic but is one which varies considerably from individual to individual and from race to race.

On the social side, the extent to which an individual can call on group support and the strength of these from the extended family, nuclear family or friends will clearly be of considerable importance.

Restated and summarised the foregoing three hypotheses can be set out as follows: health changes which are dependent upon the presence of other members of the same species will not be universal – affecting all people in the same manner and with the same disorders.

The consequences will be dependent on: (a) the importance of the relationships that become disordered; (b) the position of the individuals experiencing such disordered relationships in the status hierarchy; (c) the degree to which the population under study has been unprepared by previous experiences for this particular situation, in other words, has had insufficient time to adapt, and (d) the nature and strength of available group supports that could have a protective function.

The conclusion from the evidence is that variations in group relationships and of the individual within the group rather than having a specific aetiological role for a particular disorder will enhance disease susceptibility in general. The disorder that emerges will be influenced by the genetic predisposition of individuals and the nature of the physicochemical or microbiological insults they encounter. Some further evidence favouring this concept of a generalised susceptibility has been provided by CHRISTENSON and HINKLE [13] in an industrial study in the US in which they have shown that managers in a company who, by virtue of their family background and educational experience, were least well prepared for the demands and expectations of the executive industrial life – had the highest rates of all diseases, major as well as minor, physical as well as mental, long-term as well as short-term.

Studies of other disorders including tuberculosis [21] have shown that the highest rates of the disease were found in 'marginal' people, people who, for a variety of reasons were deprived of meaningful social contact. This included ethnic minorities rejected by the dominant majority, people with high sustained rates of mobility or broken family life. A similar set of circumstances have been described in the case of certain other disorders including schizophrenia [22], multiple accidents [23], suicide [24], alcoholism and non-tuberculosis respiratory diseases. The relevance of these hypotheses and concepts and the question of migration and physical illness will next be reviewed taking certain specific disorders as examples, hypertension, coronary heart disease, asthma and bronchitis.

Hypertension

The fact that a number of populations have been studied where blood pressure shows little or no increase in level with age can be taken as evidence that such changes are not an inevitable part of aging and must represent the effect of environmental factors acting over a period of time [25]. The wide range of isolated traditional groups who fall into the low pressure category make it most unlikely that genetic factors are playing a key part. Studies in people of the same broad ethnic groups living at different stages of exposure to westernised life style, have shown a considerable gradient between the groups with the more acculturated and westernised groups showing a steeper rise of blood pressure with age and a much higher prevalence of hypertension.

Low pressure populations are characterised by the smallness and cohesiveness of their societies and their relative insulation from western and industrialised cultures. Data have been reported from almost every continent including part of Africa, Asia, the Americas, Australia, New Guinea and the Pacific Islands [26].

The impact of westernised patterns of living and the effect this can have on blood pressure level can be illustrated by the higher blood pressures found in Polynesian people of Rarotonga in the Southern Cook Islands compared with the lower pressures found among atoll dwelling Pukapukans in the Northern Cook Islands, also Polynesians [27]. There are other differ-

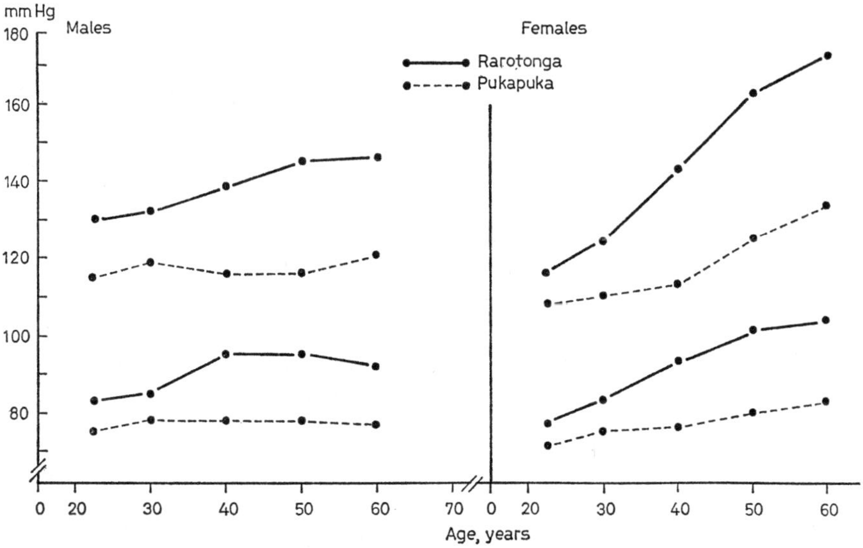

Fig. 1. Mean blood pressures in Rarotonga and Pukapuka in the Cook Islands.

ences between the groups of importance including higher mean weights in the Rarotongans, but after controlling for weight their pressures are still notably higher than the Pukapukans. The low salt appetite and salt use of the Pukapukans is an additional factor which is believed to be important. They have daily 24-hour sodium outputs of around 50 mEq compared with 120 mEq in Rarotonga. This is a highly significant between-population difference but no within-population differences in relation to sodium output and blood pressure were noted.

The changing salt use forms an important difference that migrants from isolated Pacific Islands undergo as they move into more westernised societies and could be one of the more important changes.

The comparison of blood pressures from Rarotonga and Pukapuka are set out in figure 1.

A study of blood pressure and diabetes in the Kingdom of Tonga carried out in 1973 in collaboration with the Department of Health of the Kingdom and the Pacific Regional Office of WHO has shown differences in extent of hypertension between subjects who had lived in Nuku'alofa, the main centre of the group, for at least 5 years, compared with subjects living a traditional village subsistence economy on the island of Foa in the Ha'apai group. The town dwellers had higher systolic blood pressures with more increase with age while the village dwellers had lower pressures and showed an increase only in those aged 55 and over. The extent of definite and probable hypertension using WHO criteria in the town dwellers was significantly higher than in the traditional group, p 0.001 in males and p 0.05 in the females.

The town dwellers were heavier than the traditional village dwellers but after controlling for weight the differences still remain and are significant in the majority of age groups.

In addition, lower urinary sodium concentrations were also found in the traditional group compared with those in Nuku'alofa.

The tempo of change is gradual in Tonga and it would be an exaggeration to describe those in Nuku'alofa as highly westernised in their life style but they are moving in that direction and changes following the gradient seen in other groups are present [28].

Pacific Polynesian Migrations

The migration of Polynesians from the Central and South Pacific to New Zealand took place around the 13th and 14th centuries. Their exposure to Europeans and their way of life commenced in the early part of the 19th century, and this has accelerated in tempo particularly in the 20th century. Their more recent migration has been from rural areas into towns, and this has been mainly since the mid-1940s.

Data now available from mortality statistics indicates that they have a notably higher mortality ratio from hypertensive heart disease than the European New Zealanders, particularly in the females where it is 6–10 times higher in 35–44 age groups. Going with this is a 3–4 times higher death ratio from coronary heart disease in Maori compared with European females. Greater degree of obesity, higher rates of smoking and diabetes are factors probably playing a part in this higher risk status. Psychosocial factors have not as yet been explored.

Prevalence Data for Hypertension from the Pacific

The aged standardised prevalence of borderline and definite hypertension by WHO criteria among five different population samples in the South Pacific and New Zealand, are set out in table I. This illustrates clearly the extent of the differences that may be found in four Polynesian groups

Table I. Blood pressure categories age standardised rates per 1,000

	Males		Females	
	borderline hypertension	definite hypertension	borderline hypertension	definite hypertension
N.Z. Maori	243.4	287.6	201.6	317.6
N.Z. Europeans	241.8	265.9	208.7	224.9
Rarotonga	242.5	343.4	231.9	365.7
Pukapuka	74.4	46.6	76.4	82.3
Tokelaus (1968)	102.5	79.7	152.2	151.2

living in different environments, two atoll dwelling, Pukapuka and the Tokelaus, two more westernised groups, Rarotonga and New Zealand Maori and a New Zealand European sample [27].

A study of hypertension in 50-to 59-year-old age group in Melbourne, Australia [29] has shown that hypertension was less frequent in Italian-born immigrants of both sexes compared with Australian-born subjects. The rate of those with diastolic pressures 100 mm Hg or more was 22.2% for the Melbourne, Australian-born compared with only 6.3% of the Melbourne, Italian-born subjects. The Italian-born came from Southern Italy where blood pressure levels have been found to be relatively low, and it is likely that the migrant entered Australia with lower pressures than comparable aged Australians. This again illustrates the need to define the characteristics of the migrant prior to migration.

Tokelau Island Migrant Study a Longitudinal Study

The differences in blood pressure pattern described in the different Polynesian groups in these studies were by the same observers using the same techniques for blood pressure recording and hopefully overcomes objections raised concerning difficulties of standardisation, and validity of comparisons between different groups.

The opportunity arose in 1966 to establish a prospective study of atoll dwelling Tokelau Islanders migrating from their traditional, cohesive, highly organised society to the urban milieu of New Zealand [8]. An earlier health survey in 1962 had included blood pressure measurement which suggested that the group fitted into the low pressure group with only minor increase with age. The Tokelau Islands consist of three small atolls with a very limited available land mass 8–10° south of the equator and 480 km northeast of Western Samoa.

In 1966 when the population was 2,000 a major hurricane drew the attention of the New Zealand Government to their overcrowded condition in the islands and the limited opportunities for development. A New Zealand dependency with rights of New Zealand citizenship, a resettlement programme was established aiming to bring both single young adults and families to New Zealand. Over the years prior to 1966 considerable migration had taken place from the Tokelaus to Western Samoa, with smaller numbers going to New Zealand and Hawaii [30]. In 1966 there were an estimated 500 Tokelauans in New Zealand, around the same number in Western Samoa and 2,000 living in the Tokelaus. Since that time migration has taken place from the Tokelaus under the Government Resettlement Programme and also as a result of chain migration of the pull type supported by money supplied by migrants to members of their family. Over the same period an increasing number of Tokelauans from Western Samoa have moved down to New Zealand. A register of all Tokelauans in New Zealand and in the home islands was established in 1970, and there are now 2,000 in New Zealand including infants and children, while the population in the Tokelaus has fallen to around 1,560, and that in Western Samoa to 200.

The total study population comprises all those Tokelauans in the two places – New Zealand and the Tokelaus – and comprises 3,560 subjects. The study has from the outset been established as a multidisciplinary study with a strong behavioural science component seeking to test specific hypotheses relating to the process of adaptation and the physical, social, cultural, and psychological changes associated with the migration process.

Detailed baseline medical and sociological data has been collected in the Tokelaus in 1968 and 1971 and migrants have been examined following arrival in New Zealand. In 1972 and 1973 all Tokelauans in New Zealand were examined including those who had come to New Zealand on their own initiative or with funds and support from their families already settled in the country. Over the same period detailed sociological questionnaires were administered to adults in New Zealand. The study therefore has certain important advantages compared with many migrant studies. Firstly, a large number of the migrants, both adults and children, have been examined on their home islands prior to migration and in many cases before they knew they would migrate. This has allowed examination of the characteristics of 'migrants' and nonmigrants. Secondly, the prospective medical and sociological study of those remaining on their home islands and those in New Zealand allows the rate and direction of changes to be looked at in the two very contrasting environments. Thirdly, a further advantage that will provide information on the part played by genetic and environmental factors is the documentation of detailed genealogies, going back many generations, on computer file. This will allow estimates of the heritability of different medical variables and enable examination of subjects with varying degrees of relationship in the two environments over a period of time, some in the Tokelaus and some in New Zealand.

The two competing sets of hypotheses that are being tested seeking to identify the environmental factors responsible for the changes in blood pressure patterns can be stated as follows: the one set includes a series of physical factors; calorie intake, physical activity and the associated body build and salt intake, may contribute to low blood pressure. The alternative set holds that much of the phenomenon can be accounted for by psychosocial factors; low blood pressures occurring in societies with a coherent value system which remains relatively unchallengend and unchanged during the lifetime of the oldest inhabitants.

The Tokelau study offers a valuable opportunity to look at these hypotheses and to help sort out whether one or other or perhaps a combination of diet, salt and degrees of adaptation of the migrant to his needs in the new society are important in the determination of blood pressure levels.

The emphasis on this type of study in this review is justified by the major contribution hypertension makes to disease, and by the fact that research up until the present has made so little headway in sorting out the factors contributing to changing pattern of blood pressure with age and its concomitant problems.

Baseline Results

The results of the initial baseline examination carried out in the Tokelaus in 1968 have been published [8, 28, 31] and show that the Tokelauans are a low pressure group, but do show some increase in blood pressure with age which is less than is found among Rarotongans and New Zealand Maori. Their body weight and body mass patterns also approximate closely to the New Zealand Maori and they are significantly heavier than the Pukapukans.

Data on the characteristics of the migrants prior to migration has been obtained, based on the 1968 survey in Tokelau [8]. Premigrant status was

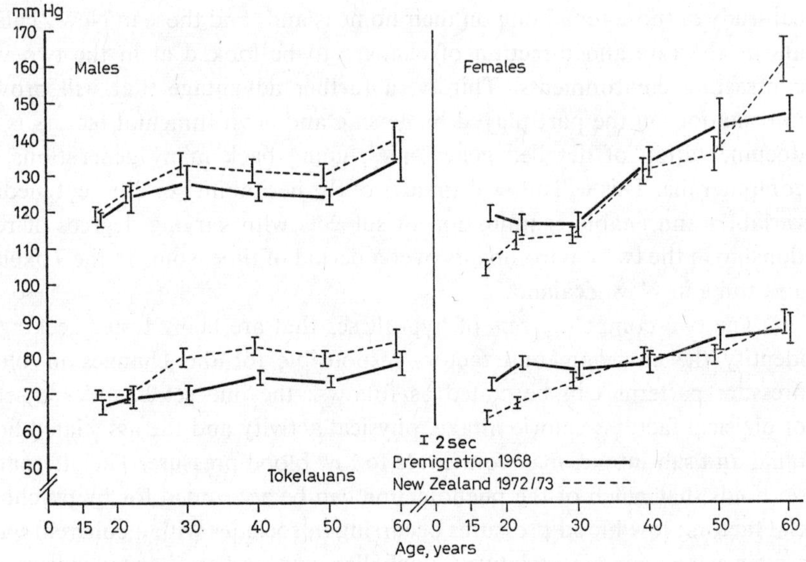

Fig. 2. Blood pressure of male and female Tokelau migrants prior to migration and after periods of up to 5 years in New Zealand.

assigned to those examined in the islands in May 1968 who migrated to New Zealand between May 1968 and August 1973. Those who remained on the islands are classed as nonmigrants. The male premigrants tend to be slightly taller and heavier than nonmigrants. Systolic and diastolic blood pressures were higher in the younger male premigrants but not in the older. Female premigrants did not differ in systematic fashion from the nonmigrants. Few of the differences in the males reach conventional statistical significance. On the other hand, the findings may suggest a selective process whereby the younger and more athletic males are the active initiators of migration, while the females and older males who migrate tend to do so in response to the decision made by the younger males and for this reason show no difference from the nonmigrants.

The prospective study has been underway since 1968 and so the trends of blood pressure, weight and other variables can now be examined in subjects who were seen on their home islands prior to migration and have been examined again after periods of up to 5 years in New Zealand. The results are group data, and are preliminary but nevertheless show some interesting trends.

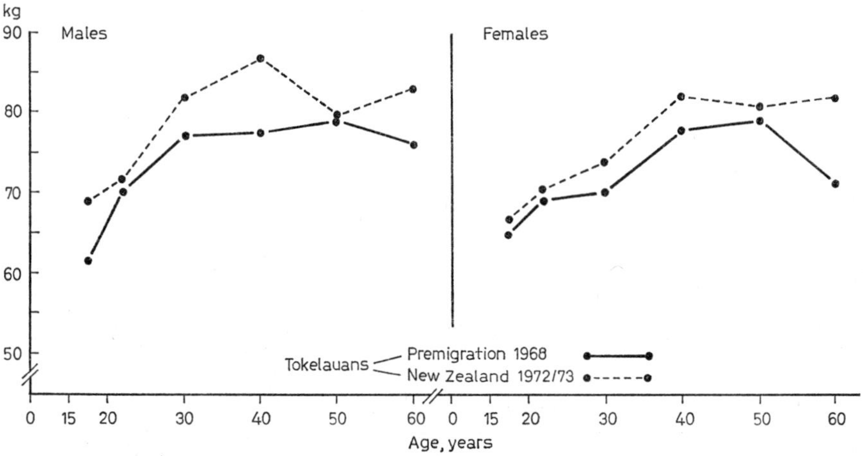

Fig. 3. Mean weights in kg of male and female Tokelau migrants prior to migration and after periods of up to 5 years in New Zealand.

The blood pressures in the males are tending to rise while the females show no change (fig. 2). The weights of both sexes are higher in New Zealand than they were on their home islands (fig. 3). The cholesterol and uric acids show no changes while the triglycerides and the casual early morning urinary sodium concentrations are very much higher (fig. 4, 5).

The dietary data being collected confirms a much higher intake of refined carbohydrate and sugar in the migrants in New Zealand, and a much greater use of salt.

Blood Pressure and Social Interaction

The specific hypotheses relating to the way in which psychosocial factors may contribute to changes in blood pressure and hypertension are now being tested.

A 'social interaction score' has been developed from the sociological questionnaire [32]. This has proved an effective measure of interaction with New Zealand institutions and Europeans during work and leisure times as compared to those subjects, who, even in New Zealand, are still primarily living and working almost entirely with other Tokelauans, attend their own Pacific Island churches and clubs. The exciting results coming forward indi-

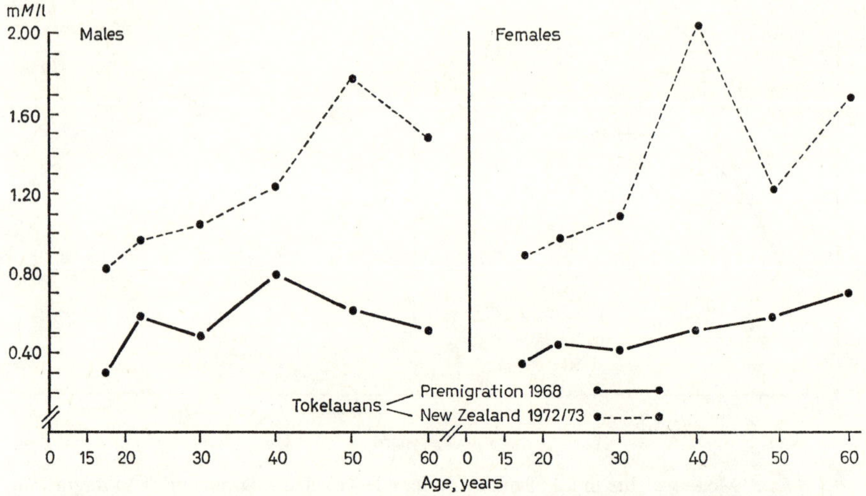

Fig. 4. Mean triglycerides in mM/l of male and female Tokelau migrants prior to migration and after periods of up to 5 years in New Zealand.

cate that the systolic blood pressure and extent of definite and borderline hypertension is significantly higher in both males and females in those at the high interaction or European end of the scale compared with those who are low interactors and are primarily mixing and involved with Tokelauans. The differences in systolic pressure are still significant after correction of blood pressure for age changes by z scores. It is clear that body mass changes, and length of stay in New Zealand could intervene in both the blood pressure and interaction variables. Using partial correlation coefficients, increasing systolic and diastolic pressures in males and females are associated with an increase in New Zealand interaction and this was not a consequence of body mass variation or of length of exposure to the New Zealand way of life.

This certainly supports the first hypothesis that the migration experience itself with the social changes, culture conflict, and lack of feedback are having a greater effect in those at the European end of the interaction scale. The development of the longitudinal file will allow more critical analysis and answer the question as to whether the European interacters had higher blood pressures prior to migration.

Other studies which show changes in migrant populations compared with those still living in their traditional self-contained settings include those carried out on Easter Islanders by CRUZ *et al.* [33]. He found in two

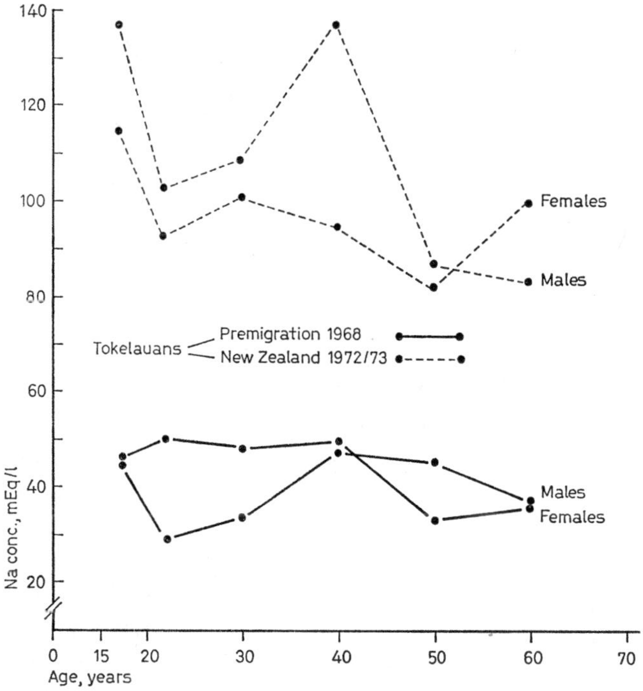

Fig. 5. Mean casual early morning urinary sodium concentrations in mEq in male and female Tokelau migrants prior to migration and after periods of up to 5 years in New Zealand.

groups, identical in terms of genetic markers, that the blood pressures of the urban group were higher in each succeeding age group whereas those in the traditional rural area showed no such change.

Coronary Heart Disease

One of the most valuable studies describing the different extent of coronary heart disease (CHD) and coronary heart risk factors in persons of the same ethnic group in three distinct environments is the Japan, Hawaii and California heart study of men of Japanese descent. The study was set up by the National Heart and Health Institute and has been in progress since 1965 [34, 35]. A gradient has been shown with mortality and prevalence of CHD increasing from Japan to Hawaii to California.

Comparing the three population groups, similarity has been found between the indigenous and migrant populations in such characteristics as blood groups and other measures representing primarily genetic influences. Differences have been noted in the diet and in smoking habits, reflecting primarily cultural influences and differences have also been noted in weight, blood pressure, glucose tolerance and in serum lipid and uric acid levels, these characteristics being dependent presumably on a varying mixture of genetic, cultural and environmental influences.

The prevalence of hypertension was highest in California, intermediate in Japan and lowest in Hawaii. Angina pectoris was more prevalent in California but differences in the prevalence of Q wave abnormalities indicating myocardial infarction were not statistically significant. Among men dying and coming to necropsy, the Hawaii descendants showed an increased frequency of CHD manifestations compared to those in Japan. This Hawaiian preponderance using standardised procedures and criteria was fourfold for severe coronary artery atherosclerosis, nearly twofold for old myocardial infarction and five- to sixfold for acute myocardial infarction.

A study in the Hawaiian cohort has shown that serum cholesterol, blood pressure, relative weight; uric acid and cigarette smoking stand out as risk factors for the development of CHD. Glucose intolerance and measures of physical activity were not so associated nor was an association shown between dietary fat and coronary risk.

Differences in saturated fat do not completely explain the serum cholesterol differences between the cohorts, nor do differences in serum cholesterol, blood pressure and smoking explain the differences observed in CHD prevalence between California and Japan. Recently, MARMOT and SYME have examined whether the striking cultural and social differences between the Japanese in Japan and in California could be contributing to the CHD difference [35]. It was predicted that those Japanese Americans who were most acculturated to a western way of life would have a higher prevalence of CHD than those whose culture is more traditionally Japanese.

To test this, 3,809 Japanese Americans in the San Francisco Bay area were examined and classified according to degree of acculturation to western culture. Those Japanese Americans who were least acculturated, who adhered more to traditional Japanese family customs and food use had a low prevalence of CHD approaching the low levels seen in Japan. More acculturated Japanese had a prevalence of coronary disease approaching the high levels seen among other Americans. Analysis showed that this difference was not due to differences in diet, smoking habits, blood pressure, serum cholesterol, serum triglycerides or serum glucose. The important conclusion put forward by these workers was that a culture characterised by strong social supports, stability and lack of individual competitiveness may be protective from CHD. This clearly supports the Cassel hypothsis relating to how protective factors may function in migrants.

Israeli Migrant Studies

Studies in Israel have made many important contributions in the field of migration and physical disease, including CHD. Full documentation of these would require an extensive review that will not be attempted. Varying prevalences of manifestations of CHD have been shown with lower rates in those from oriental countries compared with those from eastern and central Europe. Few of these studies have included examination of migrants prior to migration [36]. The Ischaemic Heart Disease Project involving 10,059 male government and municipal employees examined in 1963, 1965 and 1968 has brought forward most valuable prevalence and incidence data [37]. The highest rates were in those from eastern and central Europe, while those from the Middle East and North Africa were significantly lower. The infarct incidence rates were higher in the first generation Israeli compared with those immigrants from the same country of origin but were substantially lower for second generation subjects. These results could indicate protective factors still operating in the migrants which become less in the first generation group, or alternately that environmental factors take a longer period to cause their effect.

An Australian Contribution

Further valuable data is available from Australia on the way in which environmental rather than genetic factors contribute to the emergence of CHD [38]. Native born Australian whites have a mortality from arterio-sclerotic and degenerative heart disease of 169/100,000 over the age range 40–49 years. Italians resident in Australia for up to 6 years have a mortality of 16/100,000 at the same age; however, with 7–19 years of residence this rises to 51/100,000 and with more than 20 years residence it is 130/100,000. A similar increase in ischaemic heart disease mortality has been shown in United Kingdom, Norwegian and Irish immigrants to the United States.

These examples in the area of hypertension and CHD have shown how migrant studies are contributing to knowledge of some of the major cardiovascular problems. Important questions arise as to whether sufficient insight can be gained to not only help in the prevention of these disorders in those areas where they are major problems, but more hopefully to limit the development and extent of these in those countries where the rate and occurrence is now starting to increase [28].

Chest Diseases Including Asthma

There is some evidence indicating that the migrant particularly coming from the tropics is at particular risk for acute and chronic chest infections particularly bronchitis. The increased material affluence that they achieve in their new society is associated with greater use of tobacco and this plays an important part in contributing to risk and chronicity of chest infections [39].

The poor housing, overcrowding and difficulty in coping with acute upper respiratory infections all play their part in both a higher rate of pneumonia but also contribute to development of chronic bronchitis.

In the area of chronic bronchitis, studies carried out by REID [40] have been most valuable. They have shown that the British have an excess of serious chronic bronchitis morbidity compared with British who had migrated to the USA. Current cigarette smoking and air pollution were considered to be important factors contributing to the differences. The age adjusted death rates from chronic nonspecific lung disease also showed considerable differences between the British in the United Kingdom, British in the USA, and US born in USA. The mortality and morbidity rates are set out in table II. This can be cited as an example where some aspects of the migrants health experience improves following migration.

Table II. Mortality from chronic nonspecific lung disease and morbidity (persistent cough and phlegm) rates in native British and US residents and in migrant group

	Death rates/100,000		Morbidity rates, %	
	males	females	males	females
British in UK	125	24	19	8
US born in USA	24	4	11	4
British in USA	23	4	8	3

Asthma

In a series devoted to psychosomatic disorders it is fitting that the final condition considered should be asthma which has so often been regarded as of psychosomatic origin.

Studies in Israel have shown that immigrants are at high risk for asthma, probably through environmental allergies and psychological stress [41]. Different Jewish ethnic groups differ in their predisposition to asthma. The great variety of climates in Israel has a notable influence on those with seasonal asthma. Seasonal variation in pollens, mould spores have also been identified and are important in some cases. A review of asthma in the Tokelau Island Migrant Study has shown that this disorder is extremely uncommon in these Polynesian people living on their home islands [42].

The limited atoll environment, the absence of many factors such as industrial pollutants and chemicals, the extremely limited availability of dairy products such as milk and butter may all contribute to this. Certainly the picture is very different among the migrants shifting to New Zealand where this disorder occurs much more frequently and is often disabling, causing loss of time from work and requiring continuous medication. The relative risk of asthma is 18.7 times greater in Tokelau males and 4.4 times greater in Tokelau females in New Zealand compared with those in the Tokelau Islands [43]. Among infants and children in New Zealand a higher rate of eczema as well as asthma has focussed attention on the fact that almost all children are breast fed for 6–10 months on the home islands, whilst in New Zealand the period of breast feeding is becoming shorter and infants and children are being exposed to unprocessed milk protein and products that they have never had before. This may well provide a potent allergic stimulus and thereby contribute to the problem.

In the adult a whole range of extrinsic allergies could be of importance ranging from housemites and fungi to industrial agents.

The linking of medical and sociological questionnaire data seeking to assess the process of adaptation and stress will enable examination of the scores of those with and without asthma to be compared.

Conclusions

A discussion on migration and physical illness poses poblems because the data available is limited in its extent, and because it is basically difficult data to collect unless a real effort is made to establish the base population on which rates can be based. The migrant arriving in his host country will become eligible for health insurance in those countries where such systems operate and his records will be merged with the records of the general population in doctors' practice files, in health insurance and hospital records. The answer must lie in special studies where information is collected in the following areas:

(1) Demographic data to provide the data base of the group being studied.

(2) Epidemiological data concerning health and disease including morbidity and mortality.

(3) Environmental data documenting the type and extent of changes in a whole range of areas including diet, living and working conditions.

(4) Social and cultural changes and there the study must involve a profound knowledge of the structure, organisation and ethnology of the migrants parent community as well as the changes that occur as they settle and adapt or fail to adapt to the social and cultural aspects of the host society. The adaptive mechanisms and strategies need documentation by skilled behavioural scientists and cannot be expected to be properly appraised by medical personnel on their own.

It must be stressed that studies of this type can only be properly undertaken by bringing together a multidisciplinary team with skill in the areas of medicine, epidemiology, biostatistics and the behavioural sciences including demography, sociology and anthropology. The orientation of different studies will vary depending on the questions being posed and the hypotheses being tested. The Cassel hypotheses as set out certainly gain support from the initial results of the Tokelau Island Migrant Study and from the Japanese California results reported by MARMOT and SYME. At the same time migrant studies must continue to document and test as far as possible the influence of environmental factors. In the area of hypertension this must include information on body weight change, diet and salt use, glucose handling, tobacco and alcohol use. It could be argued that the changes related to the experience of migration itself, the social uprooting, culture conflict and lack of feedback would have a more immediate effect that would lessen with adaptation compared with environmental factors such as diet change, salt use and weight gain. This needs to be tested further in long-term migrant studies, including information concerning migrant status prior to migration. The concept of protective factors, both social and biological is an important one and properly developed may allow for more effective intervention than attempts to reduce 'stressor' situations.

The contribution of genetic factors particularly in the control of biological responses to migration has been attempted in some studies such as those of CRUZ in Chile, by collection of specific genetic markers. The Japan Hawaii California study controls for genetic factors simply by taking people of the same broad ethnic group. The Tokelau Island Migrant Study offers further opportunities to look critically at the genetic environmental interaction with the migrant population in urban, industrialised New Zealand, and those remaining in Tokelau in a very different environment. Given the opportunity, support, and funding, properly planned studies of the migrant, migration and adaptation should be scientifically rewarding and help produce knowledge that could not be gained in any other way. The important fact stands out that the application of the knowledge already available could lessen very considerably many of the health hazards that the migrant and his family face and this certainly constitutes a challenge to the community and to those concerned with preventive medicine.

Acknowledgements

The author wishes to acknowledge the support of the Medical Research Council of New Zealand, the Cardiovascular Disease Unit of the World Health Organisation, the Wellington Hospital Board and the Department of Health in the studies relating to the Epidemiology Unit research programme detailed in this paper.

References

1 MORRIS, J.N.: Four cheers for prevention. Proc. R. Soc. Med. *66:* 225–232 (1973).
2 BLACK, I.A.; LEWIS, H.E.; THACKER, C.K., and GOULD, A.K.: Tristan de Cuhna: general medical investigations. Br. med. J. *ii:* 1018–1024 (1963).
3 RAVENSTEIN, E.G.: The laws of migration. J.R. Stat. Soc. *48:* 167–227 (1885).; reprinted in the BOBBS-Merrill report series No. 5 482.
4 United Nations: Multilingual demographic dictionary. English section. Pop. Stud. No. 29 (New York 1958).
5 United Nations: Methods of measuring internal migration. Pop. Stud. No. 47 (New York 1970).
6 KOSINSKI, L.A. and PROTHERO, R.M.: People on the move. Studies on internal migration (Methvan, London 1975).
7 MABOGUNJE, A.L.: Systems approach to a theory of rural-urban migration. Geogr. Anal. *2:* 1–18 (1970).
8 PRIOR, I.A.M.; STANHOPE, J.M.; EVANS, J.G., and SALMOND, C.E.: The Tokelau Island Migrant Study. Int. J. Epidem. *3:* 225–232 (1974).

9 SELYE, H.: The stress of life (McGraw-Hill, New York 1956).
10 DUBOS, R.: Man adapting, pp. 164-165 (Yale University Press, New Haven 1965).
11 CASSEL, J.C.: Physical illness in response to stress; in LEVINE and SCOTCH Social stress, pp. 189–209 (Aldine, Chicago 1970).
12 SYME, L.: Cultural mobility; in FEJFAR WHO report on cardiovascular epidemiology in the Pacific, p. 51 (1970).
13 CHRISTENSON, W.W. and HINKLE, L.E., jr.: Differences in illness and prognostic signs in two groups of young men. J. Am. med. Ass. *177:* 247–253 (1961).
14 RAHE, R.H.: Subjects' recent life change and their new future illness susceptibility. Adv. psychosom. Med., vol. 8, pp. 2–19 (Karger, Basel 1972).
15 HENRY, I.P.; MEEHAM, J.P., and STEPHENS, P.M.: The use of psychosocial stimuli to induce prolonged hypertension in mice. Psychosom. Med. *29:* 408–422 (1967).
16 SCOTCH, N.A.: Sociocultural factors in the epidemiology of Zulu hypertension. Am. J. publ. Hlth *52:* 1205–1231 (1963).
17 SYME, S.L.; HYMAN, M.M., and ENTERLINE, P.E.: Cultural mobility and the occurrence of coronary heart disease. Hlth hum. Beh. *6:* 173–189 (1965).
18 SYME, S.L.; BORHANI, N.O., and BUECHLEY, R.W.: Cultural mobility and coronary heart disease in an urban area. Am. J. Epidem. *82:* 334–346 (1965).
19 STAMLER, J.; BERKSON, D.M.; LINDBERG, H.A.; MILLER, W.A.; STAMLER, R., and COLLETTE, P.: Socioeconomic factors in the epidemiology of hypertensive disease; in STAMLER, STAMLER and PULLMAN The epidemiology of hypertension, pp. 289–320 (Grune & Stratton, New York 1967).
20 CASSEL, J.C.: The relation of the urban environment to health. Towards a conceptual frame and a research Strategy in migration and related social and health problems in New Zealand and the Pacific; in STANHOPE and DODGE Proceeding of a Seminar, Wellington 1972, pp. 119–131 (1974).
21 HOLMES, T.: in SPARER Multidiscipline studies of tuberculosis in personality, stress and tuberculosis (International Univ. Press, New York 1956).
22 MISHLER, E.G. and SCOTCH, N.A.: Sociocultural factors in the epidemiology of schizophrenia. A review. Psychiatry *26:* 315–351 (1963).
23 TILLMAN, W.A. and HOBBS, G.E.: Social background of accident-free and accident repeaters. Am. J. Psychiat. *106:* 321 (1949).
24 DURKHEIM, E.: Suicide (Free Press, New York 1957).
25 HUIZINGA, J.: in VORSTER Casual blood pressure in populations in human biology of environmental change, pp. 80–86 (IBP, London 1972).
26 CASSEL, J.C.: Hypertension and cardiovascular disease in migrants. Int. J. Epidem. *3:* 204–206 (1974).
27 PRIOR, I.A.M.: Cardiovascular epidemiology in New Zealand and the Pacific. N.Z. med. J. *80:* 245–252 (1974).
28 The prevention and control of cardiovascular disease. Rep. Sem. Regional Office of World Health Organisation for the Western Pacific, Manila 1975.
29 LOVELL, R.R.H. and PRINEAS, R.J.: The identification and treatment of hypertensives in two Australian urban communities. Int. J. Epidem. *3:* 26–29 (1974).
30 HOOPER, A. and HUNTSMAN, J.: A demographic history of the Tokelau Islands. J. Polyn. Soc. *82:* 366–411 (1973).

31 PRIOR, I.A.M.; HOOPER, A.; HUNTSMAN, J.; STANHOPE, J.M., and SALMOND, C.E.: The Tokelau Island Migrant Study. Case study prepared for Human Adaptability Section of the International Biological Programme; in AINSWORTH HARRISON Population structures and human variation (Cambridge University Press, London, in press).
32 PRIOR, I.A.M.; CASSEL, J.C.; HOOPER, A.; HUNTSMAN, J.; SALMOND, C.E.; STANHOPE, J.M., and BEAGLEHOLE, R.: Blood pressure patterns in polynesian migrants. A study of the effect of social interaction and migration on blood pressure levels. Tokelau Island Migrant Study (in preparation).
33 CRUZ, C.; ETCHEVERRY, R., and NAGEL, R.: Influence of migration on blood pressure of Easter Islanders. Lancet *i:* 697–699 (1964).
34 KAGAN, A.; HARRIS, B.R.; WINKELSTEIN, W., jr.; JOHNSON, K.G.; KATO, H.; SYME, L.S.; RHOADS, G.G.; GAY, M.L.; NICHAMAN, M.Z.; HAMILTON, H.B., and TILLOTNOW, H.: Epidemiologic studies of coronary heart disease and stroke in Japanese men living in Japan, Hawaii and California. Demographic, physical, dietary and biochemical characteristics. J. chron. Dis. *27:* 345–364 (1974).
35 MARMOT, M.: Social and cultural factors in coronary heart disease in Japanese Americans; in STANHOPE Proceedings of a seminar: Migration and Health, Wellington 1975, pp. 57–77 (1977).
36 DREYFUSS, F.: Epidemiology of cardiovascular disease in Israel; in ELIAKIM and NEUFELD Cardiology current topics and progress, pp. 56–61 (Academic Press, London 1968).
37 MEDALIE, J.H.; KAHN, H.A.; NEUFELD, H.N.; RISS, E.; GOLDBOURT, U.; PERLSTEIN, T., and ORON, D.: Myocardial infarction over a five year period. 1. Prevalence, incidence and mortality experience. J. chron. Dis. *26:* 63–84 (1973).
38 SHEPHERD, R.J.: The influence of race and environment on ischaemic heart disease. Can. med. Ass. J. *111:* 1336–1340 (1974).
39 SEMPLE, A.B.: The health and care of immigrants. R. Soc. Hlth J. *2:* 96–99 (1967).
40 REID, D.D.: Bronchitis among the British. Israel J. med. Scis *7:* 1569–1572 (1971).
41 GLAZER, I.: Etiologic factors in bronchial asthma in Israel. Int. Archs. Allergy appl. Immun. *36:* 172–179 (1969).
42 STANHOPE, J.M. and PRIOR, I.A.M.: The Tokelau Island Migrant Study. Prevalence of various conditions before migration. Int. J. Epidem.
43 STANHOPE, J.M.: The Tokelau Island Migrant Study. Prevalence of common conditions in atoll and N.Z. dwellers compared; in STANHOPE Proceeding of a Seminar, Wellington 1975, pp. 99–109 (1977).

Dr. I. PRIOR, Director, Epidemiology Unit, Wellington Hospital, *Wellington* (New Zealand)

Adv. psychosom. Med., vol. 9, pp. 132–139 (Karger, Basel 1977)

Occupational Mobility and Health

EMIL BERKANOVIC and PAMELA C. KROCHALK

School of Public Health, University of California, Los Angeles, Calif.

Contents

The impact of social change on health has been of considerable interest to health researchers. Indeed, the consequences of change have been studied from a number of points of view. Some researchers have sought correlations between social change of any sort and subsequent changes in health status, assuming that various changes, although differently weighted, have a simple additive effect on health [e.g. 13, 14]. Other researchers have examined the relationship between specific types of social change assumed to be problematic for individuals and changes in health status [e.g. 15, 20].

One type of change the health implications of which have been extensively studied is social mobility. Social mobility refers to any change in the social circumstances under which a person lives. Such changes may occur intergenerationally between the family into which the individual was born and his present life, or they may occur intragenerationally between some past time in the individual's life and the present. Further, social mobility is a multidimensional construct referring to a wide range of changes that may or may not accompany each other.

Geographical mobility is one such dimension. Studies in this area may seek correlations between intragenerational geographical changes and health, or they may examine differences in health status among dispersed groups of individuals in the same generation whose parents were born in a different specific geographic area. For example, KAGAN *et al.* [6] found mean differences in height, weight, blood pressure, and serum cholesterol among Japanese living in Japan, Hawaii, and California, all of whose parents were born in Japan.

Another dimension of social mobility is cultural mobility. SYME *et al.* [18] defined cultural mobility as a change in the 'cultural scene' or 'social world' such that an individual experiences incongruities in customs, values and beliefs. Such changes may accompany geographical mobility on the part of the individual or they may result from social changes occurring in a given locale. Although cultural mobility and geographic mobility are often viewed as two aspects of a common process, there are examples where the effects of cultural mobility may be assessed independently of changes in geography. For example, TYROLER and CASSEL [20] have studied the impact of urbanization on rates of coronary heart disease among residents of a formerly rural county suffering from urban sprawl.

Yet another dimension of social mobility is status mobility. It is this dimension upon which the present paper is focused. Mobility of status refers to changes in the social ranking of an individual. Since education, occupation, and income are the common indicators of social status, changes in any of these may be taken as evidence of status mobility. For several reasons, however, this paper will be restricted to an analysis of research bearing on occupational mobility and health. First, BLAU and DUNCAN [1] have shown that status derived from occupation is highly intercorrelated with status derived from education and income. Thus these indicators are interchangeable. Second, assuming that change affects health through the creation of incongruous experiences, changes in occupation would appear to be the most directly relevant indicator of status mobility. Third, and most persuasive, there has been little research on status mobility in which educational or income changes have been used as the indicators. What follows, then, is a review and discussion of the research bearing on occupational mobility and health.

The Effects of Occupational Mobility on Health

Literature on occupational mobility and health was obtained by means of a multistage search. First, computer assistance in the form of the MEDLARS system was used in order to retrieve any entries in *Index Medicus* for the 4 years immediately prior to the search. Then, the tables of contents of a number of journals in which relevant research was likely to have been published were examined over a 10-year period. Finally, the bibliographies of all research reports retrieved were examined for references to additional research.

There are four generalizations that can be made about this literature.

(1) There are surprisingly few studies that bear directly on the relationship between occupational mobility and health.

(2) The vast majority of the research on this topic is confined to coronary heart disease.

(3) Most of the research focusing on this topic fails to control for the effects of the other types of social mobility that usually accompany occupational mobility. Thus, even where an unequivocal association between occupational mobility and health can be established, it is necessary to distinguish such effects as geographic and cultural mobility that may accompany changes in job status before causal significance can be attributed to this association.

(4) Most studies fail to control for the joint effects of initial and destination status on any relationships observed between occupational mobility and health. As a consequence, such relationships may be more parsimoniously explained as the result of differences in the expected additive effect of the two statuses. This is a problem where there is evidence suggesting status differentials in the distribution of a particular disease.

Intragenerational Effects

Four studies were found in which intragenerational occupational mobility was shown to affect health. KAPLAN *et al.* [7] reported an increase in coronary heart disease among those respondents in the two lower social classes who were upwardly mobile as compared with the nonmobile population. Upward mobility among the upper social classes, on the other hand, appeared to be protective. That is, a significantly lower rate of coronary heart disease was found among the upwardly mobile than among the nonmobile in the upper classes. While KAPLAN *et al.* offer no explanation for this finding, they suggest that the upper classes are better socialized for successful adaptation to new life styles than are their lower-class counterparts who lack appropriate preparation and social supports and who may, therefore, find the mobility experience more stressful. Finally, they also suggest that occupational mobility may have an independent effect among the lower socioeconomic stratum in addition to the effect of status. Unfortunately, they do not present data bearing on this issue.

KASL and COBB [8] examined the impact of forced unemployment, an elemental form of occupational mobility, on the blood pressure levels of industrial workers experiencing layoff. Blood pressures were found to be high during the periods of anticipated layoff, unemployment, and the probationary period following reemployment. They returned to normal, however, once reemployment was established. The same authors show similar findings for changes in cholesterol and serum uric acid levels [9]. Since changes in the blood pressure, cholesterol and uric acid levels of individuals were the dependent variables in these studies, the impact of unemployment cannot be confounded with other status differentials. Nor were other forms of social mobility at issue.

SYME *et al.* [19], in a study conducted in North Dakota, found higher rates of coronary heart disease among the occupationally and geographically mobile than among the nonmobile. SYME *et al.* [17] also found similar results in a study in California. Further, these relationships held after body weight, diet, cigarette smoking and parental longevity were controlled.

Several other studies, however, found that intragenerational mobility had no impact on health. HINKLE *et al.* [3] examined prospectively the relationship between changes in job status in a large corporation and the incidence of coronary heart disease. Based on data for a 5-year period, they concluded:

> The findings provide no evidence that men who have high levels of responsibility, or who have been promoted rapidly, frequently, or recently, or men who are transferred to new departments or to new companies, have any added risk of coronary heart disease. On the other hand, men who enter the organization with a college degree have a lower attack rate, death rate, and disability rate for coronary heart disease at every age, in every part of the country, and in all departments of the organization. The difference in risk appears to exist at the time the men are hired and apparently is not greatly changed by any of the subsequent experiences of the men (p. 245).

These findings support those reported in several previous studies in which relationships between changing levels of responsibility and coronary heart disease were explored. LEE and SCHNEIDER [10] studying male employees in the oil industry, found the highest incidence of arteriosclerotic disease among nonexecutives in dead-end jobs. Similarly, PELL *et al.* [12] in a longitudinal study of 90,000 employees of Du Pont Company representing five levels of economic status and job responsibility, suggest an inverse relation between job level and incidence of myocardial infarction. MORTENSON *et al.*

[11] found little difference in coronary death rates between management and laborers. Similarly, WHITNEY [23] found no relationship between promotions and death from coronary heart disease among men employed by the Bell System. Taken together, these studies fail to support the hypothesis that organizational advancement and increased responsibility add to the risk of coronary heart disease.

Intergenerational Effects

Three studies were found in which intergenerational occupational mobility was related to the incidence of coronary heart disease. BRUHN *et al.* [2] found a slight relation between these variables in comparing a sample of coronary patients with a control group matched for age, sex and social class. SHEKELLE *et al.* [16] found a positive relationship between intergenerational status mobility and coronary heart disease among a broad spectrum of employees in a major utility company. Subjects whose class of origin was different from their present social class had a relative risk of CHD of 1.5. Those experiencing changes of three levels or more had over twice the risk of CHD than men moving a fewer number of levels.

KAPLAN *et al.* [7] in a study previously mentioned with respect to intragenerational mobility, also found some evidence for a relationship between intergenerational mobility and coronary heart disease. Paralleling their findings with respect to intragenerational mobility, they found that the intergenerationally mobile among the lower classes were also at higher risk of heart disease than were the mobile among the upper classes.

Two studies were found in which no relationship was reported between occupational mobility and health. WARDWELL *et al.* [22] and WARDWELL and BAHNSON [21] studied two separate samples of men with first myocardial infarctions and compared them with a randomly chosen control group matched for sex and age. In neither study was there evidence of a link between either intergenerational or intragenerational occupational mobility and the illness.

Conclusion

It appears, then, that the evidence regarding occupational mobility and health is both thin and equivocal. Indeed, considering the problem of confounding occupational mobility with other forms of mobility, one may well ask whether the effects of occupational mobility *per se* can ever be isolated. Further, assuming that such isolation is at least technically possible, there remains the question of the practical significance of such an analysis, given that the vast majority of the occupationally mobile are also mobile in a myriad of other ways.

Perhaps the most sophisticated discussion of this issue is contained in SYME *et al.* [18]. Working within the rubric of cultural mobility and breaking that concept into several components – generational, career, residential and situational – they found that the relationship between occupational mobility and coronary heart disease is a function of many of these components in interaction. These data would suggest, therefore, that one ought not expect to find a simple relationship between occupational mobility and health, and that any relatiohships that do appear are probably suggestive of a particular experience with respect to the components of cultural mobility.

At a minimum, attributions of the effects of occupational mobility ought not be made without first taking into account the simpler effects of initial and destination status. For example, although two of the studies previously discussed, BRUHN *et al.* [2] and SHEKELLE *et al.* [16] concluded that there was a relationship between intergenerational mobility and coronary heart disease, HORAN and GRAY [4] reanalyzed each using the following formula:

$$B = a + b_1X_1 + b_2X_2 + b_3I(X_1, X_2),$$

where X_1 = initial status, X_2 = destination status, and $I(X_1, X_2)$ = the mobility effect.

This reanalysis showed that less than 1% of the variance in the SHEKELLE *et al.* data, and that less than 2% in the BRUHN *et al.* data could be attributed to mobility *per se.*

Thus, at present there is very little evidence in support of a relationship between occupational mobility and health. Further, in a recent study carried out among a large sample of six American communities, JACKSON an CURTIS [5] found no statistically significant evidence of a relationship between occupational mobility and a broad spectrum of variables that have been postulated to be affected by mobility. Linking these findings to a methodologically critical review of previous research, these authors conclude that there is little evidence in support of any hypothesis in which status mobility is the independent variable. HORAN and GRAY's reanalysis add further support to this position.

In conclusion, the work of SYME *et al.* [17] suggests that a rather complex set of relationships may exist between the social mobilities and health.

It is possible that none of these situations taken alone or together constitute a relevant parameter, but they really are reflections of a significant but ill-understood process. Following this reasoning, occupational mobility...and other similar sociocultural factors may only be reflections of a significant process which has not yet been delineated and studied (p. 345).

Indeed, an understanding of these processes requires a more sophisticated formulation of the independent variable than that suggested by the title of this paper.

References

1 BLAU, P. and DUNCAN, O.J.: The American occupational structure (Wiley, Chichester 1967).

2 BRUHN, J.; CHANDLER, B.; MILLER, C.; WOLFE, S.; LYNN, T., and BIRD, H.: Social aspects of coronary heart disease in a Pennsylvania German community. Soc. Sci. Med. *2:* 201–212 (1968).

3 HINKLE, L.; WHITNEY, L.; LEHMAN, E.; DUNN, J.; BENJAMIN, B.; KING, R.; PLAKUN, A., and FLEHINGER, B.: Occupation, education, and coronary heart disease. Science *161:* 238–246 (1968).

4 HORAN, R. and GRAY, B.: Status inconsistency, mobility and coronary heart disease in an urban area. J. Hlth soc. Behav. *15:* 300–310 (1974).

5 JACKSON, E. and CURTIS, R.: Effects of vertical mobility and status inconsistency. A body of negative evidence. Am. sociol. Rev. *37:* 701–713 (1972).

6 KAGAN, A.; HARRIS, B.; WINKELSTEIN, W.; JOHNSON, K.; KATO, H.; SYME, S.; RHOADS, G.; GAY, M.; NICHAMON, M.; HAMILTON, H., and TILLOTSON, J.: Epidemiologic studies of coronary heart disease and stroke in Japanese men living in Japan, Hawaii and California. J. chron. Dis. *27:* 345–364 (1974).

7 KAPLAN, B.; CASSEL, J.; TYROLER, H.; CORNONI, J.; KLEINBAUM, D., and HAMES, C.: Occupational mobility and coronary heart disease. Archs. intern. Med. *128:* 938–942 (1971).

8 KASL, S. and COBB, S.: Blood pressure changes in men undergoing job loss. A preliminary report. Psychosom. Med. *32:* 19–38 (1970).

9 KASL, S. and COBB, S.: Changes in serum uric acid and cholesterol levels in men undergoing job loss. J. Am. med. Ass. *206:* 1500–1507 (1968).

10 LEE, R. and SCHNEIDER, R.: Hypertension and arteriosclerosis in executive and nonexecutive personnel. J. Am. med. Ass. *167:* 1447–1450 (1958).

11 MORTENSON, J.; STEVENSON, T., and WHITNEY, L.: Mortality due to coronary heart disease analyzed by broad occupational groups. Archs. ind. Hlth *19:* 1–4 (1959).

12 PELL, S.; D'ALONZO, C., and ANTHONY, C.: Acute myocardial infarction in a large employed population. Report of a six-year study of 1,356 cases. J. Am. med. Ass. *185:* 831–838 (1963).

13 RAHE, R.; MCKEAN, J., and RANSON, A.: A longitudinal study of life-change and illness patterns. J. psychosom. Res. *10:* 355–366 (1967).

14 RAHE, R. and PAASIKIVI, J.: Psychosocial factors and myocardial infarction. A pilot study. J. psychosom. Res. *15:* 19–24 (1971).
15 SCOTCH, N.: Sociocultural factors in the epidemiology of Zulu hypertension. Am. J. pub. Hlth *53:* 1205–1213 (1963).
16 SHEKELLE, R.; OSTFELD, A., and OGELSBY, P.: Social status and coronary heart disease. J. chron. Dis. *22:* 381–394 (1969).
17 SYME, S.; BORHANI, N., and BUECHLEY, R.: Cultural mobility and coronary heart disease in an urban area. Am. J. Epidem. *82:* 334–346 (1966).
18 SYME, S.; HYMAN, M., and ENTERLINE, P.: Cultural mobility and the occurrence of coronary heart disease. J. Hlth hum. Behav. *6:* 178–189 (1965).
19 SYME, S.; HYMAN, M., and ENTERLINE, P.: Some social and cultural factors associated with the occurrence of coronary heart disease. J. chron. Dis. *17:* 277–289 (1964).
20 TYROLER, H. and CASSEL, J.: Health consequences of cultural change. II. The effect of urbanization on coronary heart mortality in rural residents. J. chron. Dis. *17:* 167–177 (1964).
21 WARDWELL, W. and BAHNSON, C.: Behavioral variables and myocardial infarction in the Southeastern Connecticut Heart Study. J. chron. Dis. *26:* 447–461 (1973).
22 WARDWELL, W.; HYMAN, M., and BAHNSON, C.: Socio-environmental antecedents to coronary heart disease in 87 white males. Soc. Sci. Med. *2:* 165–183 (1968).
23 WHITNEY, L.: Coronary heart diseases among men in the Bell system. J. occup. Med. *10:* 14–20 (1968).

Dr. E. BERKANOVIC, School of Public Health, University of California, *Los Angeles, Calif.* (USA)

P.C. KROCHALK, Doctoral Candidate, School of Public Health, University of California, *Los Angeles, Calif.* (USA)

Adv. psychosom. Med., vol. 9, pp. 140–159 (Karger, Basel 1977)

Retirement and Physical Health

FRANCES M. CARP
The Wright Institute, Berkeley, Calif.

Contents

The word 'retirement' is used to denote three quite different phenomena: an event, a process, and a status [15]. Physical health is related complexly and in different ways to each of the three. Health is often given as a reason for retirement ending the work career, and here plays the role of determinant of the event, the date of the 'gold watch dinner'. Physical health affects the retirement process which goes on within the individual over a period of time both prior to and following the retirement day, a conscious or unconscious working through of adaptation to different demands, the transition from the status of adult producer to that of elderly consumer. One major influence on all aspects of life style during the several life stages after the work career has been completed is health. Many observers believe that the process and status of retirement, in turn, affect physical health, though they do not agree whether that effect is beneficial or detrimental.

First we will consider some of the evidence regarding health as a causal factor in regard to retirement, then, some regarding retirement as an influence upon physical health.

Impact of Health on Retirement

In considering the effects of physical health on retirement, it is useful to make a further distinction between retirement as an institution, a social function, versus retirement as an event, a process and a status or stage in the life of a person [74]. Health is often offered as the major rationale for retirement, both by employers and policy makers in explaining the institution and by retirees in announcing their personal decisions. However, the percentage of individuals who cite health as the reason for their retirement varies, depending upon the date of data collection and upon the conditions under which the response is obtained, suggesting that 'poor health' may sometimes be a face-saving answer [47]. On the institutional side, retirement policies and practice use chronological age, not health, as the basic criterion of retirement readiness [8]. Moreover, the rate of retirement of older workers rises disproportionately when there is any increase in unemployment [32], which suggests that economic pressure is important in putting the older worker at a disadvantage, and that 'retirement due to ill health' may be a euphemism for job loss and continued unemployment. Yet the impact of health problems upon personal decisions to end the work career is real. Men who leave the labor force, giving the reason of health, are less likely to move back into it when economic conditions become more favorable [67].

The Role of Health in the Decision to Retire

Estimates regarding the prevalence of health problems as causal to individual decisions to retire vary widely. For example, in a nationwide survey conducted by the United States Bureau of the Census in 1952, 60% of the men aged 65 and older out of the labor force said health was the reason they retired [68]: according to data from a national sample in 1957, 40% of men and of women 65 and over said they retired due to ill health [64]; while a study using Census data from 1967, 1968 and 1969 found ill health the reason for retirement among only 18% of men in that age bracket [32]. At least some of that wide difference in national figures reflects changes in health status, retirement policy and benefits, and attitudes toward retirement during the intervening years.

Several variables complicate the issue. Type of work performed is one. THOMPSON and STREIB [69], who concluded from their study that poor health is a common cause of retirement, also found it most frequent among blue-collar workers. Similarly, STEINER and DORFMAN [68] observed that few professional workers, compared to those in lower level jobs, cited health as reason for leaving the labor force. Age is another complication. JAFFEE [32] found 'ill health' the leading reason given for their retirement by men in the 45–64 age bracket, the 'early retirees', though not among those 65+.

From these and other studies it seems clear that men in good health tend to remain in their jobs longer, and that 'early retirees' tend more often to mention health. However, men who retire at 65 or later not only tend to have better health, they also tend to be better educated, to hold higher level (and more interesting and well paid) jobs, and to be white. Education, job level and race/ethnicity are also related to retirement age [32, 49]. The better educated and whites, as well as those in higher level jobs, tend to have longer work careers. Given this matrix of interrelated predictive variables, it is difficult to assess the exact role of physical health in determining retirement date.

Most retirement investigations have been concerned with men [31] and only recently is there growing interest in retirement patterns of women [30]. However, it is apparent that sex differentials will be found to interact with other factors such as job level in affecting the relationship between health and the decision to retire. Analyzing data from a community sample, SPENCE [66] observed a sex difference in retirement which may largely reflect a difference in health. Among early retirees, the men were more likely to say they had been forced to retire while the women were more likely to consider themselves voluntary retirees. Like JAFFE, SPENCE found health mentioned as the reason for retirement much more often by early retirees (nearly three-fourths of the youngest age group), and almost twice as many men as women in this age group were perceived by their interviewers to have at least a mild health problem. Sex then joins education, job level and race/ethnicity in confounding the relationship between health and retirement age.

The situation is further complicated by the fact that early retirement usually involves the penalty of reduced payments under private pension plans and Social Security, and perhaps a hiatus before benefits begin. Both individuals and production suffer because some individuals must, for financial reasons, work to normal retirement age despite failing health or physical impairment.

How many individuals retire because they are doing poor work because of poor health? How many who do not retire are ill and are only waiting for their pensions to become available? They struggle on, while their work has a deleterious effect on their health [20].

On the other hand, many older people need to work not only to provide income but also in order to maintain a balance of 'deep-seated personality needs that have been satisfied by certain environmental conditions to which they have grown accustomed and upon which they have become highly dependent' [38]. Such individuals are frequently denied these opportunities because of retirement regulations or hiring restrictions. These policies and practices are often based upon the assumption that the health of older people, as a group, is such that continued employment is not feasible.

The Health Status of Older Adults

Some studies question this conclusion and indicate that, while the incidence of chronic or disabling diseases is higher for the aged than for the young, the health status of most older adults is reasonably good.

In the National Health Survey of 1957, most older people reported they were not limited in their activity or mobility [64]. Only 10% of people 65 years of age and older said they were unable to carry on their regular work and only 7% were unable to go outside without help. About 83% of persons 45–64 reported no chronic condition or limitation of activity. At the ages of 65 and above, problems increased, but still the majority (nearly 58%) reported they were without chronic condition or limitation. From these data it appears that those with long-term disability or chronic ailment are but a minority of the older population. KUTNER *et al.* [38] conclude:

...in view of the emphasis on the poorer health status of the old, as compared with the young, we perhaps need to be reminded that millions of persons past middle age consider themselves to be in reasonably good health and capable of performing useful tasks in our society.

Somewhat later, ROSENFELD and WALDMAN [58] concluded similarly from a review of the literature that 'very large numbers' of men aged 65 and older consider themselves in sufficiently good health to work, since in some studies half the men aged 65 and older reported no chronic condition which limited or prevented work activities. Similarly, the report from a special committee of the Gerontological Society [26] summarized the evidence to conclude that the large majority of persons beyond retirement age are not limited by illness or disability. In a Massachusetts survey [60] most retirees (85%) reported 'good' or 'very good' health, although 32% indicated some limitation imposed by their health and 40% had made more than routine visits to a doctor. Among TIAA/CREF beneficiaries, only 7% considered their health 'poor' [50].

However, opinion is conflicting. Reviewing the evidence, EISDORFER [21] comments on: 'The remarkably high proportion of older persons suffering from chronic diseases' and cites OSTFELD's [53] study of old-age assistance recipients, among whom physicians found the incidence of disease to be 'appalling'.

Self-Evaluation versus Medical Assessment of Health

One major source of confusion in describing the health of older people is that various studies have defined health differently. In most, physicians' examinations have not been available, and health data have largely been respondents' self-evaluations and those of the interviewers, usually supported by checklists of ailments and questions regarding such somewhat more objective matters as frequency of medical attention and days in bed. There is evidence that self-perceptions of health have some basis in fact [64]. However, serious pitfalls in using self-estimation of health to make judgements about physical status have been identified [20]. If health is to be used in deriving implications about functional capacity [40] and to separate illness from age, it must be more accurately defined.

Unfortunately, medical examinations usually are out of the question in research on retirement, primarily because of cost and also because of possible invasion of privacy. When medical data are available on samples of older people, they diverge widely from self-evaluations and suggest a much higher rate of illness and incapacity.

In a study of Old Age Assistance recipients in Cook County, Illinois, it was apparent, from looking at what people said about their health and health practices, that they did not view themselves as unwell. 'However, when we come to what physicians find in detailed histories, workups, electrocardiograms, etc., we see a different picture and a startling paradox. The prevalence of major illnesses in this population as seen by physicians is staggering' [53]. The old people saw themselves as not being in particularly bad shape, but physicians were 'horrified' by the widespread, serious illness. For instance, 3 in every 4 of these people should have been taking medication every day for such disorders as diabetes, high blood pressure and parkinsonism.

OSTFELD's was a very special sample, among whom incidence of disease would be unusually high while health care practices would be poor and medical attention not a lifetime habit. However, among a sample of community volunteers who underwent 2 days of examination at Duke University Medical Center, about one-third of the aged significantly misjudged their physical condition [12]. SHANAS *et al.* [65], who used an index of functional incapacity to compare with self-evaluations of physical ability to work concluded that, among retired men they classified as having no incapacity, almost 3 in each 10 said their health was too poor for them to work.

There is urgent need for better definition of what constitutes health among older people. No accurate estimate of the health status of old people in general, let alone explication of the relationships between health and retirement, is possible without it. The available evidence suggests that, in addition, older people need to be educated to distinguish conditions which can and should be treated from 'old age', which must simply be borne.

Health as Reason for Retirement as Institutionalized

Poor health as characteristic of older people is frequently cited as society's reason for creating the institution of retirement. 'First of all, retirement exists in the expectation that persons beyond a certain age will suffer a chronic loss in fitness or capacity so that they will be unable to continue to work effectively' [8]. Other reasons are to provide a reward for long years of hard work and contribution to production, and the need to provide access to jobs for younger persons (who also work for less pay). If poor health is a primary reason for institutionalizing retirement, why is health status not used as a direct criterion of readiness to retire? In terms of health, one person may be ready for retirement at 45, and another not yet ready at 70, but in practice, health status is rare as a retirement policy guide.

Results of medical examinations are not quite as objective – and not nearly as inexpensive – as birthdates, and not all jobs have the same requirements or demands for physical health, but if consideration for health is a major determinant of the social policy of retirement, adequate criteria can be developed which relate health status and disabilities to job requirements. An index of health status more relevant to retirement than time since birth would be valuable not only out of consideration to individuals who object to age-arbitrary retirement rules, but also so that society may benefit from the capabilities of healthy persons of whatever ages.

It is unlikely that such an index will be used. Administrators find it easier to deal with clear-cut standard rules, and age is nicely objective and impersonal. Another consideration is that 'failing' a health examination might be a traumatic documentation of worthlessness to the individual. Arbitrary rules based on age have a significant advantage: the person forced to retire can blame 'the system'. Development of screening batteries would be expensive and time-consuming because they would have to be based on special job-analyses and would be different from job to job. Perhaps most impotant, this approach to retirement on a policy level would limit the effectiveness of retirement in balancing the labor force and insuring access to jobs for young persons.

Concurrent retirement age changes and changes in the nature of work do call into question the justification of retirement policies through reference to health, as significantly more rational than reference to age. Mechanization and automation have reduced physical effort and work hours. At the same time, people have been retiring at younger and younger ages. KREPS [37] has demonstrated that if current trends continue, normal retirement age in 1985 might be 39. It has been officially predicted in Great Britain that by the late 1970s only about 7% of men aged 65–69 will remain at work. Failing health may have been a central consideration when retirement age was more nearly coincident with death, and work was physically arduous. As retirement age moves down and medical care improves, there should be reconsideration of the extent to which health is a reason or rationalization for retirement policy.

Impact of Retirement on Health

There is a persistent belief in our society that there is a relationship between retirement and subsequent decline in health. Some experts point to retirement as the 'greatest killer of the mid-sixties': some studies find no consistent effect of retirement on health; and still others indicate that retirement is beneficial to physical well-being.

Deleterious

According to a report of the American Medical Association Committee on Aging [1]: 'Medicine sees in retirement a direct threat to the health and life expectancy of the persons affected'. BORTZ [10] writes of 'retirement shock, well known to physicians', and comments that masked suicides are not rare. It is a common saying that 'medical miracles can prolong life threatened by illness, but no one has yet found a cure for retirement'. Summarizing the literature, KENT [35] finds a set of conjectures associated with retirement which predict negative effects including physical deterioration.

ELLISON [22] proposes that the 'sick role' may sometimes be adopted as preferable to the 'retiree role'. The rationale is that retirement is identified with hopelessness and helplessness, while the sick are expected to recover. Also the sick role seems more consistent with the dependent or at least non-producer status retirees have.

JOHNSON [33] includes somatic complaints in a 'retirement syndrome' which also includes depressive affect and social withdrawal, and he relates this reaction to unresolved conflicts centered around the loss of work and around increased difficulties in interpersonal relationship with spouse, family and others. SHANAS *et al.* [65], in a discussion of the common perception of retirement as a loss, and the consequent reaction of depression, comment that, 'the relation of depression to physical illness is critical. The depressed person usually has a number of specific physical symptoms', and note that, 'the physician often treats these as if they were «typical problems of old age»'.

In trying to understand what might be causal links between retirement and health decrements, it is helpful to consider some of the components, attributes or correlates of retiring. For one thing, at retirement income typically is 'chopped in half' [59]. One direct effect is curtailment of funds for health care and medical attention. At retirement, a large proportion of people are, for the first time, reduced to incomes below the poverty level [11].

The incidence of poverty is highest among the elderly, of all population segments [11]; and the official 'poverty line' is lower for the old than for the young, and even lower for old women than for old men [52]. Even for those with 'good' retirement incomes, relative deprivation in economic terms is almost universal – relative to their own life-long incomes and relative to the purchasing power of the general market.

Furthermore, work usually means more to an individual than mere subsistence. His job provides a bond between the worker and his community. Work is a social function, creating a sense of belongingness. Working validates self-esteem. The values society teaches us to cherish most highly – self-reliance, achievement, contribution to family and society – are the very ones retirement threatens. One's very identity may seem to be lost as he leaves gainful employment and faces the threat of dependent idleness.

Another major concomitant of retirement is sudden expansion of 'free time' with its many problematic consequences [36]. According to MARTIN [43], one of the earliest psychiatric recognitions of the problem of free time was FERENCZI's description of the 'Sunday neurosis' in 1919. Some of FERENCZI's patients developed nervous conditions which recurred regularly on days of rest. The syndrome included what FERENCZI [23] called 'little hysterical symptoms', including headaches, depression, gastrointestinal symptoms, and oversleeping. According to BUTLER [13]: 'One not uncommonly sees such phenomena in association with retirement.'

Considering the variety and the pervasive nature of the new demands retirement places upon the person, that process may reasonably be assumed to involve, for many if not all persons, a period of stress and, moreover, of multiple stress. The many studies of relationships between stress and disease (for example, those of SELYE [63] and of LEVI [41]) have documented the intimate relationship between the endocrine glands and the central nervous system, and have demonstrated measurable changes in endocrine function, due to stress, which may affect a variety of organs and organ systems. BORTZ [10] points out that the evidence is particularly clear with regard to the heart and blood pressure, and that a large proportion of adult deaths result from breakdown of the heart and blood vessels to the brain and other parts of the body. There is an extensive literature documenting effects of environmental or situational variables upon blood pressure and other cardiovascular functions [25]. Much of this literature deals with transient responses to experimentally induced stimuli, but some studies report more or less persistent cardiovascular changes following the occurrence of significant life events confirming clinical observations [54, 57, 62, 72, 73].

Development of techniques for quantifying life events in terms of their health impacts has accelerated over the past few years [2, 5, 34, 39, 46, 61, 71]. Two of the best known are the Schedule of Recent Experiences [27], and the MRFIT (multiple risk factor intervention trial) *Inventory of Life Events* [51]. The technique has proven its usefulness as a predictor of a variety of illnesses, in both retrospective and prospective studies [19].

One of the more important considerations, from the point of view of the impact of retirement upon physical health, is that the recent life events *need not be negative,* in and of themselves, in order to be predisposing to physical illness. Various life events are of greater and lesser significance, and attempts are made to represent this difference in terms of numeric 'weights', as is recency [28]. The important point, for the present discussion, is that *change* in conditions and behaviors is the central predictive factor.

One item in both scales mentioned above is 'retirement from work'. However, due to the nature of retirement, most people who check this item must also check a number of other 'life events' listed in either inventory. Some common examples are: a major change in eating habits, not being able to do things you used to because of age, a change in your usual level of physical activity (at work as well as during leisure time), success and/or awards at work, fewer responsibilities, fewer hours at work, a major career decision, quitting your job, becoming more involved in hobbies or sports, the realization that you will never attain an important goal, a difficult decision, being worried about financial security, a personal decision which alienated you from your friends, separation from a close friend, fewer social contacts than before, change in group social relationships, financial difficulties, a change in your personal habits (dress, friends, life-style, etc.), a vacation, and change of the status of the family within the community. Many other items must be checked by a large proportion of honest retirees; these represent only the items which seem almost universal in the retirement process. They comprise a significant portion of the 147-item MRFIT Inventory.

In summary, there is considerable opinion and some evidence that retirement may have negative consequences for physical health, and there are several possibilities for the mediation of this effect. One is the decimated income which may necessitate reduced health and medical care; another is the 'Sunday syndrome' reaction to the '7-day week-ends'; still another is the depression which accompanies the experience of retirement as an ego threatening loss; and perhaps the most inclusive, the fact that the occurrence of multiple changes or 'life events', whether good or bad, is predictive of physical illness.

The more major the change and the larger number of 'life events', the greater the likelihood of physical illness. Retirement is not one event, process, or condition, but a complex matter which affects all facets of life. On this basis, retirement should often precipitate physical illness. Even if leaving work and the attendant changes in the conditions and style of life are desired and favorably perceived by the retiree, the sheer scope and pervasiveness of *changes* must forecast physical illness, according to the Holmes and Rahe paradigm. Studies are needed to test this hypothesis, and they must be designed in view of the many confounding variables which obscure the overall meaning of the literature on health and retirement.

Beneficial

Some studies suggest that retirement is salutary rather than deleterious to physical health. For example, while 10% of a sample of Massachusetts retirees reported poorer health postretirement, nearly a quarter reported improved health [60]. In MULANAPHY's [50] 1974 study, 32% of the people who reported that they retired due to poor health now evaluated their health as 'good' or 'very good'. THOMPSON and STREIB [69], who found poor health a frequent cause of retirement, particularly among blue-collar workers, also found that their health might well improve following retirement. MARTIN and DORAN's [44] 1967 survey data on men over 55 show a steadily increasing incidence of illness requiring medical attention, which drops from 50 to 30% immediately after retirement. They interpret this as indicative of a reduction in illness.

Other interpretations are, of course, possible. As workers, these men may have had medical attention available on the job. A suspicious observer might suggest that some workers 'call in sick' on days of major baseball games and the like, while retirees do not. On the other side, in some blue-collar work a relatively minor ailment may interfere with work, and require 'days off sick', but when staying at home in retirement one would put up with more discomfort before seeing a doctor. This might be particularly true in view of reduced income.

Awareness of some ailments is less when the individual is at rest than when he is involved in sustained physical activity at work. EISDORFER [21] points out that early or mild forms of many chronic diseases are rarely observable until the victim exerts himself. Cardiovascular illness and emphysema, common disorders among older people, may manifest themselves initially only as shortness of breath upon exertion. A retired person may exert himself less, experience fewer symptoms, and therefore report his health improved. His physician might or might not agree. There are counter biases in that the benefits of retirement may not be readily observed by persons with subtle and minor physical problems. The research data are simply not conclusive.

In the absence of clear-cut studies, the incidence of poor health as an effect of or adaptation to retirement may be overestimated because physicians tend to see the ill, and other service personnel to deal with 'at risk' retirees. The same bias is clear in research. For the investigator, observation of retired persons in institutions, treatment centers or service agencies is tempting because of their visibility and availability. Yet it is the normal person in the population at large who is of greatest importance. One weakness in the fund of knowledge concerning retirement is the tendency to study unusual groups of old people [14, 64]. Indeed, research in the behavioral sciences generally suffers distortion because investigators must collect data on people who are available to them [17]. Retired persons who are financially insolvent, ill or poorly adjusted come to the attention of the community and are more likely to be available as subjects for studies. It is hazardous to generalize from these findings. The decisive information regarding interactions of health and retirement must include data on community-resident respondents who do not self-select into the study through some unusual dependency or identification with an elite group.

> Perhaps the stress which some contend is placed by retirement upon physical health reflects the concern of physicians, psychiatrists, and medically oriented researchers whose experience is mainly with sick people [48].

In the judgment of MITCHELL, who has undergone retirement as well as studying it, the negative effect of retirement upon physical health has been exaggerated: 'to suggest that the rigors of retirement adjustment will undermine physical health is largely nonsense. (We have yet to see our first case of diabetes, or even dandruff, caused by retirement.)' MITCHELL believes the chances much greater that, relieved of job pressures and having more rest, regular meals and greater freedom for pursuits he enjoys, the retiree's physical health will improve, though MITCHELL acknowledges that, 'mental health may be something else again'.

It Depends

The positive versus negative impact of retirement upon physical health is much debated. Some physicians and others who work with older people consider retirement a central trauma of the aging period [70]. BARRON [6] goes so far as to say that death comes at retirement for some. However, others who have worked with and studied older people suggest that retirement is not always unwelcome, and that adaptation to it may be favorable to physical and mental health [18, 56, 65, 70].

There is urgent need, in view of the increasing numbers of persons undergoing the process, and the extension of years in the status of retirement, to clarify the conditions in which retirement is damaging to health and those in which it is beneficial. There is some suggestive evidence.

Individuals with very little to do often lapse into hopelessness and apathy. FILER and O'CONNELL [24] compared the adjustment of retirees who worked and those who did not. The working people had better adjustment scores in the area of health as well as in those of usefulness and happiness. CARP [16] found similar advantages among old people who either worked for pay or had a regularly scheduled volunteer responsibility.

BARRON [6] posits five 'universal functions' of work: it provides income, regulates life activity, offers status or social identification, permits association with others, and makes available a meaningful life experience. If work is simply a financial arrangement, the retiree will welcome its cessation, provided he is assured of a continuing income. If work provides other 'universal functions' in his life, he may suffer 'retirement shock' which often causes aches and pains and many produce serious illness.

According to BEATTY [7] and MITCHELL [47], the retirent who did not plan ahead for this new status is the one who suffers 'retirement shock' and often becomes sick or infirm, while those who prepared seem happier and in better health.

Expectations regarding effects on health seem to condition attitudes toward retirement [45] and may well influence actual health outcomes. MITCHELL [48] suggests that the exaggerated picture painted of the casualties of retirement, which he believes to be the consequence of selective attention to the ill, itself constitutes an additional hazard for the person undergoing or facing retirement. He must *expect* to suffer physical trauma.

JACOBSON [29] found that people who wanted to retire when they reached pensionable age overwhelmingly believed retirement affects health positively. 'Conversely, work-oriented respondents tended to accept as wholeheartedly the equally stereotyped opposite view that retirement is detrimental to health.' Expectations varied also according to the degree of strain imposed by the job. Men in 'heavy' jobs tended to expect retirement to be conducive to good health, while those in 'light' jobs tended to attribute ill-effects to retirement.

The Meanings of Retirement

From individual to individual, the meaning of retirement varies widely.

> Retirement has many meanings to those undergoing it: the end of individual worth and social contact, a haven of rest, relief from an unpleasant, overtaxing or health-draining job, or completion of commitment to society and initiation of self-realization. It may

be a ceremony between one career and another; it may represent the opportunity to start one's 'real' life work or to draw two paychecks [15].

The impact of health upon retirement, and the reverse impact of retirement upon health, must be understood in terms of this variation in meaning. The timing of the retirement event, the nature of the retirement-adaptation process, and the life-style in retirement status all will be affected by the person's own interpretation of the meaning of retirement.

In the minds of already retired people, as well as those asked to look ahead to describe retirement, good health is associated with other positive descriptors. ATCHLEY [4] factor analyzed semantic differential responses and obtained four factors of attitude toward retirement among retired workers. 'Healthy-sick' appeared in the factor he labeled physical potency, which also included relaxed-tense, mobile-immobile, able-unable, independent-dependent, hopeful-hopeless. The implication is that retired workers who perceive retired people to have good health also think of them as relaxed, mobile, able, independent, and hopeful; while those who associate retirement with poor health perceive retirees as tense, immobile, unable, dependent and hopeless.

Social Changes, Historical Trends and Cohort Differences

Both the institution of retirement and characteristics of retirees are undergoing rapid and drastic change. It is only recently that the event of retirement is a normal one in the life history, that most people undergo the process, and that a large population segment lives in retirement status. That population segment is growing rapidly, as more and more people live into later adult years and as retirement age drops. Today's retirees are a pioneer generation; tomorrow's will be in many ways unlike them, and the context of retirement will be far different also.

As retirement age drops [37], physical health improves due to medical research and improved services, and additional breakthroughs seem to be on the way. For example, EISDORFER [20] suggests that surgical banks will provide artificial organs and a kind of 'youthfulness' in age: 'If we know enough about genetics to know that our kidneys will give out at 60, perhaps we can replace the organ at 45 and the weak link in the organ chain may be strengthened', and he asks: 'What, then, will be the impact of retirement upon an «active» and «youthful» individual?'

Financial considerations call into question the extent to which retired people will benefit from medical advances. OSTFELD [53] points to the incredible cost of applying existing medical care techniques to the older adult population, and the cost of such innovations as 'organ banks' cannot be low. At present, medical expenses are higher for older people. For example, in 1969, per capita medical expenses for people in this country aged 65–74 were one-third higher, and for people 75 and older, two-thirds higher than for people in the next-younger age cohort, 55–64. All are, of course, higher than for the population at large [32]. In that same year, household income for families with heads aged 65 and older was exactly half that for other households. Moreover, JAFFEE clearly documented a serious 'deterioration in the economic position of the older families' from 1950 to 1969. Continuing and even increasing economic deprivation among the retired, relative to the overall potential market for medical services, must be anticipated and has serious negative implications for the impact of retirement upon health in future years.

Meanwhile, the physical stress of work declines. The work force is increasingly in white-collar rather than blue-collar jobs, and even for the latter, physical effort is increasingly being replaced by machines. This is no doubt one reason why fewer laborers say they retire due to health problems. For example, ASH [3] found that among steelworkers in 1951 the prevalent reason for retirement was ill health, but by 1960 retirement was being justified primarily as a reward for a lifetime of work.

At all levels of society, thinking is moving from the painful prospect of retirement *from* to the more optimistic matter of retirement *to,* and considerations of the affirmative aspects of a leisure life-stage. As the work week and work year have diminished, people have increasing experience with leisure prior to the end of the work life. Increasingly there are efforts to include retirement education in curricula, and to introduce retirement preparation programs into business and industry. This experience and instruction may diminish the stress of 'time unlimited', though there remains the possibilty that tomorrow's retirees, compared to their predecessors, will show 'little improvement in knowledge of how to spend uncommitted time wisely' [55].

Summary and Implications

Health is a major factor in adaptation and satisfaction at any age, and perhaps becomes increasingly influential as disease and disorder accumulate in the later years. In relation to retirement, health is a pervasive variable that plays many roles: it is a cause of retirement and a factor in retirement policy as well as a determinant of retirement adjustment [64, 65]. In turn, it probably is affected by that adjustment [10, 48].

There is little doubt that persons of retirement age tend to have more illnesses and disabilities than younger people do. The incidence of disease and health risks among older people probably is appallingly high [53]. Physical illness is an important cause of psychiatric disorder among older people [9, 42, 66]. Yet the specific effects of health on use of leisure, and the relationship of increment of diseases and disabilities to reduction in feelings of well-being and energy as people move into retirement have not been explored adequately.

How much do feelings of well-being express medical status and how much do they reflect general satisfaction with life [14]? To what degree is satisfaction with life dependent upon physical well-being [47]? How seriously do feelings of worthlessness and hopelessness affect health status? Perceptions of health status?

Poor health as a reason for retirement is no doubt realistic in many cases; it may be euphemistic in some. On the other hand, the retiring person may present an overly optimistic view of his physical condition in order to qualify for retirement housing [14] or in other ways to maintain independence and freedom.

The area of health and retirement is an extremely complex and important one in which major research efforts should be undertaken. Health is a pervasive variable that turns up under all headings of 'retirement': it is a cause of the retirement event, a factor in retirement policy, a determinant of adaptation during the process of retiring, and of life-style subsequently; and it is effected by the nature of that process and life-style. A concerted effort should be made to clarify these relationship.

It may well be that there is no simple answer: that retirement, in and of itself, does not necessarily have either a favorable or a deleterious effect upon those who enter it. Many aspects of the person's character, education, previous occupation and life-style – as well as factors in the social and cultural surround – combine to influence the course of his health as well as other aspects of his adjustment to the changed situation.

The urgent need is for longitudinal studies which follow a cross section of people from well before to considerably after the retirement date, or even the decision to retire. These studies must include both thorough medical assessments and self-report as outcome variables; and their design must control for every one of the many confounding variables. It is a sizeable task, but only this approach will untangle the conundrum of retirement and physical health.

References

1 American Medical Association: Report of the Committee on Aging (American Medical Association, Washington 1966).

2 ANTONOYSKY, A. and KATS, R.: The life crisis history as a tool in epidemiological research. J. Hlth hum. Behav. *8:* 15 (1967).

3 ASH, P.: Pre-retirement counseling. Gerontologist *6:* 97–99, 127–128 (1966).

4 ATCHLEY, R.C.: Research studies in social gerontology. Final report on research grant 93–P–57498/6 (Administration on Aging, Washington 1975).

5 BARRABEE, P.; BARRABEE, E.L., and FINESINGER, J.E.: A normative social adjustment scale. J. Psychiat. *112:* 252 (1955).

6 BARRON, M.L.: The aging American. An introduction to social gerontology and geriatrics (Crowell, New York 1961).

7 BEATTY, R.P.: The senior citizen (Thomas, Springfield 1962).

8 BELBIN, R.M.: Implications for retirement of recent studies in age and working capacity; in CARP The retirement process (USGPO, Washington 1968).

9 BIRREN, J.E.; BUTLER, R.N.; GREENHOUSE, S.W.; SOKOLOFF, L., and YARROW, M.R.: Human aging: a biological and behavioral study. US Dept. of Health, Education and Welfare, Public Health Service Pub. No. 986 (Government Printing Office, Washington 1963).

10 BORTZ, E.L.: Beyond retirement; in CARP Retirement (Behavioral Publications, New York 1972).

11 BROTMAN, H.: Every tenth American – the 'problem' of aging; in LAWTON, NEWCOMER and BYERTS Community planning for an aging society (Dowden, Hutchinson & Rose, Stroudsburg, in press).

12 BUSSE, E.W.: Changes in thinking and behavior in the elderly. An interdisciplinary study. Paper presented at the Annual Meeting of the American Psychiatric Assn., Detroit 1967.

13 BUTLER, R.N.: The facade of chronological age. An interpretive summary; in NEUGARTEN Middle age and aging (University of Chicago Press, Chicago 1968).

14 CARP, F.M.: A future for the aged (University of Texas Press, Austin 1966).

15 CARP, F.M.: Summary and prospect; in CARP The retirement process (USGPO, Washington 1968).

16 CARP, F.M.: Differences among older workers, volunteers and persons who are neither. J. Geront. *23:* 497–501 (1968).

17 COMBS, A. and SNYGG, D.: Individual behavior (Harper, New York 1959).

18 CUMMING, E. and HENRY, W.: Growing old: the process of disengagement (Basic Books, New York 1961).

19 DOHRENWEND, B.S. and DOHRENWEND, B.P.: Stressful life events – their nature and effects (Wiley, New York 1974).

20 EISDORFER, C.: Discussion; in CARP The retirement process. Public Health Service Pub. No. 1778, pp. 97–104 (USGPO, Washington 1968).
21 EISDORFER, C.: Adaptation to loss of work; in CARP Retirement (Behavioral Publications, New York 1972).
22 ELLISON, D.L.: Work, retirement and the sick role. Gerontologist *8:* 189–192 (1968).
23 FERENCZI, S.: Sunday neurosis. Further considerations to the theory and technique of psychoanalysis (Basic Books, New York 1958).
24 FILER, R.N. and O'CONNEL, D.D.: A useful climate contribution for the aging. J. Geront. *17:* 350–352 (1962).
25 GUTTMAN, M.C. and BROWN, H.: Interaction of environmental factors and systemic arterial blood pressure – a review. Medicine *50:* 543 (1971).
26 HAVIGHURST, R.J.: A report of a special committee of the gerontological society. Research and development goals in social gerontology. Gerontologist *9:* No. 4, part 2 (1969).
27 HOLMES, T.H. and RAHE, R.H.: The social readjustment rating scale. J. psychosom. Res. *11:* 213 (1967).
28 HOROWITZ, M.J.; SCHAEFER, C., and COONEY, P.: Life event scaling for recency of experience; in GUNDERSON and RAHE Life stress and illness (Thomas, Springfield 1974).
29 JACOBSON, D.: The influence of fatigue producing factors in industrial work on preretirement attitudes. Occup. Psychol. *76:* 193–200 (1972).
30 JACOBSON, D.: Rejection of the retiree role. A study of female industrial workers in their '50's. Hum. Relat. *27:* 477–492 (1974).
31 JAFFEE, A.J.: Differential patterns of retirement by social class and personal characteristics; in CARP The retirement process (USGPO, Washington 1968).
32 JAFFEE, A.J.: Life style emeritus: tomorrow's retirement (Bureau of Applied Social Research, Columbia University, New York 1971).
33 JOHNSON, D.E.: A depressive retirement syndrome. Geriatrics *13:* 314–319 (1958).
34 KANNEL, W.B.: Role of blood pressure in cardiovascular morbidity and mortality. Prog. cardiovasc. Dis. *17:* 5 (1974).
35 KENT, D.: Aging: fact and fancy. Gerontologist *5:* 51–56 (1965).
36 KLEEMEIER, R.W.: Time, activity and leisure; in KLEEMEIER Aging and leisure (Oxford University Press, New York 1961).
37 KREPS, J.M.: The allocation of leisure to retirement; in CARP The retirement process, pp. 137–144 (USGPO, Washington 1968).
38 KUTNER, B.; FANSHEL, D.; TOGO, A.M., and LANGNER, T.S.: Five hundred over sixty (Russell Sage Foundation, New York 1956).
39 LANGNER, T.S. and MICHAEL, S.T.: Life stress and mental health (Free Press of Glencoe, New York 1963).
40 LAWTON, M.P.: Competence, environmental press and the adaptation of older people; in WINDLEY and ERNST Theory development in environment and aging (Gerontological Society, Washington 1975).
41 LEVI, L.: Sympatho-adrenomedullary responses to emotional stimuli. Methodologic, physiologic and pathologic considerations; in BAJUSZ An introduction to clinical neuroendocrinology (Karger, Basel 1967).

42 LOWENTHAL, M.F.; BERKMAN, P.L. *et al.:* Aging and mental disorder in San Francisco. A social psychiatric study (Josse-Bass, San Francisco 1967).

43 MARTIN, P.A.: The psychiatrist's role in free time and its uses; in MARTIN Leisure and mental health. A psychiatric viewpoint (American Psychiatric Assn., Washington 1967).

44 MARTIN, J. and DORAN, A.: Perception of retirement: time and season (Pilkington Research Project on Retirement, Liverpool 1967).

45 MCMAHAN, C.A. and FORD, T.R.: Surviving the first five years of retirement. J. Geront. *10:* 212–215 (1955).

46 MICHAUX, W.W.; GANSEREIT, K.H.; MCCABE, O.C., and KURLAND, A.A.: The psychopathology and measurement of environmental stress. Community ment. Hlth J. *3:* 358 (1967).

47 MITCHELL, W.L.: Preparation for retirement (American Ass. of Retired Persons, Washington 1968).

48 MITCHELL, W.L.: Lay observations on retirement; in CARP Retirement (Behavioral Publications, New York 1972).

49 MOORE, M.E.: Mortality and morbidity in the population; in RILEY and FONER Aging and society, vol. 1 (Russell Sage Foundation, New York 1968).

50 MULANAPHY, J.M.: 1972–73 survey of retired TIAA-CREF annuitants. Statistical report (Teachers Insurance and Annuity Association, College Retirement Equities Fund, New York 1974).

51 National Heart and Lung Institute: MRFIT (multiple risk factor intervention trial) Inventory of Life Events (National Institutes of Health, Washington 1974).

52 ORSHANSKY, M.: The shape of poverty in 1966. Social Security Bulletin, Dept. of HEW (1968).

53 OSTFELD, A.M.: Frequency and nature of health problems of retired persons; in CARP The retirement process (USGPO, Washington 1968).

54 OSTFELD, A.M. and LEBOVITS, B.Z.: Personality factors and pressor mechanisms in renal and essential hypertension. Archs intern. Med. *104:* 43 (1959).

55 RANDALL, O.: Some historical developments of social welfare aspects of aging. Gerontologist *5:* March (1965).

56 REICHARD, S.; LIVSON, F., and PETERSEN, P.G.: Aging and personality (Wiley, New York 1962).

57 REISER, M.F.: Life situations, emotions, and the course of patients with arterial hypertension. Proc. Ass. Res. Nerv. Ment. Dis. *29:* 870 (1950).

58 ROSENFELD, C. and WALDMAN, E.: Work limitations and chronic health problems. Mon. Labor Rev. *1967:* 38ff.

59 ROSOW, I.: Old age: one moral dilemma of an affluent society. Gerontologist *2:* 182–191 (1962).

60 RYSER, C. and SHELDON, A.: Retirement and health. J. Am. Geriat. Soc. *17:* 180–190 (1969).

61 SARGENT, H.D.; MODLIN, H.C.; FARIS, M.T., and VOTH, H.M.: Situational variables. Bull. Menninger Clin. *22:* 148 (1958).

62 SCHROEDER, H.A.: Pathogenesis of hypertension. Am. J. Med. *10:* 189 (1951).

63 SELYE, H.: The stress of life (McGraw-Hill, New York 1956).

64 SHANAS, E.: The health of older people (Harvard University Press, Cambridge 1962).

65 SHANAS, E.; TOWNSEND, P.; WEDDERBURN, D.; FRIIS, H.; MILHOJ, P., and STEHOUWER, J.: The psychology of health; in NEUGARTEN Middle age and aging (University of Chicago Press, Chicago 1968).
66 SPENCE, D.L.: Patterns of retirement in San Francisco; in CARP The retirement process (USGPO, Washington 1968).
67 STECKER, M.L.: Why do beneficiaries retire? Who among them return to work? Soc. Sec. Bull. *18:* 3–12 (1955).
68 STEINER, P.O. and DORFMAN, R.: The economic status of the aged (University of California Press, Berkeley 1957).
69 THOMPSON, W.E. and STREIB, G.: Situational determinants, health and economic deprivation in retirement. J. soc. Issues *14:* 18–34 (1958).
70 United States Senate: Testimony before the Special Committee on Aging (USGPO, Washington 1959).
71 VOTH, H.M.; MODLIN, H.C., and ORTH, H.H.: Situational variables in the assessment of psychotherapeutic results. Bull. Menninger Clin. *25:* 75 (1962).
72 WEISS, E.: Psychosomatic aspects of hypertension. J. Am. med. Ass. *120:* 1081 (1942).
73 WOLFF, H.G. and WOLF, S.: The management of hypertensive patients; in BELL, CLAWSON and FAHR Hypertension (University of Minnesota Press, Minneapolis 1951).
74 CARP, F.M.: Retirement (Behavioral Publications, Columbia University, New York 1972).

FRANCES M. CARP, Ph. D., The Wright Institute, *Berkeley, Calif.* (USA)

Adv. psychsom. Med., vol. 9, pp. 160–223 (Karger, Basel 1977)

Contributions of Social Epidemiology to Studies in Psychosomatic Medicine

Summarizing Discussion

STANISLAV V. KASL

Department of Epidemiology and Public Health, Yale University School of Medicine, New Haven, Conn.

Introductory Remarks

The task of a discussant of a series of diverse papers for which he has also served as coeditor is full of ambiguities and traps. Any criticism of organization or coverage of such a volume becomes self-criticism; avoidance of discussion of such limitations is intellectually dishonest. Revelations about obstacles in the way of producing such a volume and about better ideas and solutions which had to be aborted are self-serving; but total silence about such issues is a bit painful. Yet these dilemmas became inevitable because of the untimely death of the intended discussant, JOHN C. CASSEL, whose breath of vision and wisdom would have made for an invaluable contribution.

The present volume is intended to respond to the growing awareness of the closeness of the two disciplines, social epidemiology and psychosomatic medicine [e.g., EASTWOOD, 1975; JENKINS, 1972; LIPOWSKI, 1976]. The plan for the book was to illustrate this closeness by presenting two types of studies: those dealing with selected diseases or conditions and those investigating the health consequences of specific social events or changes. Even though it was clear that we wanted to exclude studies and approaches which did not reflect this disciplinary overlap (e.g., animal studies, laboratory experiments in psychophysiology), there was no grand master plan which had to be followed. Certain intended contributions (such as on cancer and rheumatoid arthritis) failed to materialize, for one reason or another. Other possible contributions, such as health effects of marital separation, were never sought after the initial impression that a critical mass of relevant evidence was not available.

Contributors were requested to emphasize evidence regarding 'physical' rather than 'mental' health outcomes and to adopt an epidemiologic perspective (a vague request indeed, as we shall see below). However, aside from being told about the overall plan for the proposed volume, they were given no other guidelines. The resultant contributions are illustrative; they are not exhaustive, representative, definitive, or criterial.

A Personal Overview of the Two Disciplines, with Special Attention to the Study of Social Change

It would be nice if social epidemiology and psychosomatic medicine were disciplines with easily defined content (methods, body of knowledge, metatheoretical orientation, practices) and well-recognized boundaries. Then one could draw a Venn diagram and the intersection of the two sets, representing these two disciplines, would be the focus of this chapter. However, such is not the case and all one can say with certainty is that both disciplines fall somewhere in the larger, also nebulous, domain of interdisciplinary collaboration between medicine and the social-behavioral sciences. This collaboration, of course, includes other disciplines, such as medical sociology or medical anthropology, thus further complicating the problem of disciplinary boundaries and overlap.

Dividing the whole field of social science-medicine not along disciplinary lines, but in terms of major problem areas, primary orientations or emphases, and levels of analysis, might suggest the following classification: (1) Concern with psychosocial determinants of: (a) illness or disease onset; (b) course and outcome of illness or disease (in the context of medical care, or without treatment; (c) medical care utilization, and (d) behaviors and practices with health implications (e.g., smoking, use of seat belts, adherence to medical regimen). (2) Concern with impact of health-illness on the behavior and well-being of the individual (e.g., impairment-disability, role performance) and the significant others (e.g., marital happiness, spouse's role performance). The above concerns can be expressed at different levels of analysis: (a) the individual (e.g., perception and interpretation of symptoms); (b) a dyad (e.g., barriers to doctor-patient communication); (c) the social network of significant others (e.g., legitimization of seeking treatment); (d) organizational (e.g., preventive health behavior in prepaid health maintenance organization vs. fee-for-service systems); (e) community (e.g., effects of catchmenting), and (f) societal (e.g., medicine as an institution of social control).

This classification cannot adequately express the richness and complexity of some of the current work in this field: multiple concerns, several levels of analysis, longitudinal perspective with multiple feedback loops. Nevertheless, this listing is adequate for the purpose of showing how difficult (and arbitrary) it would be to 'assign' a particular problem or topic exclusively to either social epidemiology or psychosomatic medicine.

The textbook definition of epidemiology is 'the study of the distribution and determinants of states of health in human populations' [McMAHON and PUGH, 1970; MAUSNER and BAHN, 1974; SUSSER, 1973]. Social epidemiology, SYME [1974] has suggested, may be seen as that part of epidemiology which is concerned with psychosocial determinants. However, because of the ecological orientation of epidemiology and the centrality of such concepts as agent-host-environment, or person-place-time, epidemiology has always been to a certain extent, 'social'. To some investigators, the term social epidemiology has also meant a broadening of 'states of health' or 'disease' to include health-relevant behaviors; thus these days one may be also studying the epidemiology of drug abuse or the epidemiology of smoking.

The agreement on a simple definition of epidemiology in no way indicates that there is also agreement on the scope and methods of epidemiology. Nor can it be said that some unique aspects of the 'epidemiologic method' have been identified to anyone's satisfaction. Epidemiology is applicable to clinical trials [FEINSTEIN, 1968] and to health services planning, administration, and evaluation [WHITE and HENDERSON, 1976]. Epidemiologists are commonly involved in large-risk factor detection and follow-up studies [e.g., STAMLER *et al.,* 1976], broad-based community intervention studies, such as the Stanford Three Community Study [e.g., STERN *et al.,* 1976], and in studies of such 'behavioral' issues as compliance [e.g., SACKETT and HAYNES, 1976]. As the claims of potential contributions of social epidemiology to other disciplines and fields of endeavor grow [e.g., CASSEL, 1974, 1976], so does, of course, the blurring of disciplinary boundaries. Overall, one is forced to conclude that one can neither set precise boundaries on 'epidemiologic methods' nor identify methodological approaches unique to epidemiology and not shared by some other discipline, such as social psychology, sociology, or demography.

An overview of recent developments and directions in psychosomatic medicine may be obtained by examining volumes 2 and 3 of the *Modern Trends in Psychosomatic Medicine* series [HILL, 1970, 1976], the series of articles in *Int. J. psychiat. Med.* (Vol. 5, issue No. 6, 1974, and Vol. 6, issues No. 1/2, 1975) entitled 'Current Trends in Psychosomatic Medicine', and the recent volumes of the *Advances in Psychosomatic Medicine*. LIPOWSKI [1973, 1976] has provided perhaps the most scholarly analysis and commentary on these recent trends. The hallmark of these developments is the freeing of psychosomatic medicine from intentional or unintentional doctrinaire moorings in any specific theoretical framework or specific methodology, and from any commitment to study certain diseases because they are 'psychosomatic'. Changes in health-illness are seen as multiply determined, and increasingly social-environmental factors are included, along with the more traditional biological and psychodynamic factors, in the search for a more adequate etiological picture. It is fair to characterize current studies in psychosomatic medicine as more pragmatic – what set of variables will best explain incidence of new cases of a disease or changes in health status – with an interest in low-level inductive generalizations rather than deductive hypothesis testing from full-blown psychodynamic formulations. And the studies which do address specific hypotheses tend to have broader theoretical formulations, involving a greater variety of variables and using a more diverse methodology.

LIPOWSKI [1976, p. 1] offers us a tripartite definition of psychosomatic medicine which (in addition to spelling out the characteristic approach to the practice of medicine and characteristic clinical activities) calls it 'a science of the relationships between psychological, biological and social variables as they pertain to human health and disease'. Given this definition and the comments above, it is difficult to find any essential and fundamental difference (in orientation or in methodology) between research in social epidemiology and in psychosomatic medicine. To be sure, there are differences in interests and differences in methodology or execution of studies, but it is hard to designate these criterial differences. For example, social epidemiologists are more likely to be concerned with the associations between social class or marital status and general morbidity and mortality, and to be intrigued by the inadequacy of our current attempts to explain these powerful, across the board associations [e.g., HINKLE *et al.*, 1976; SYME and BERKMAN, 1976]. On the other hand, investigators in psychosomatic medicine are more likely to be involved in what LIPOWSKI [1976, p. 4] calls 'studies of mediating mechanisms between symbolic stimuli and their physiological consequences'. As another example, one could note that studies in social epidemiology are more likely to involve population-based samples, while studies in psychosomatic medicine tend to depend more on 'samples of convenience', often of persons seeking some treatment. However, this reflects a difference in training, interests, priorities and values, not a fundamental disagreement on the role of representative samples or the logic of generalizing findings.

The growing convergence of social epidemiology and psychosomatic medicine may also be understood in terms of influences from other disciplines which have had a similar impact on both fields. For example, medical sociology has had a powerful influence with its theoretical formulations, perspectives, and bodies of data, including those involving (a) the sick role [e.g., PARSONS, 1958; TWADDLE, 1972], (b) illness behavior, perception of symptoms, and medical care seeking [e.g., MECHANIC, 1968, 1972; SUCHMAN, 1965a, b; ZOLA, 1972], (c) role of the family [e.g., LITMAN, 1974], and (d) various theoretical reformulations and extensions, such as the concept of the 'at risk role' [BARIC, 1969]. As another example, social psychology has provided a certain theoretical formulation, 'The Health Belief Model' [e.g., BECKER, 1974] which has become a useful framework within which to understand the whole spectrum of health-related behaviors labelled health behavior-illness behavior-sick role behavior [KASL and COBB, 1966] and various health-maintaining or risk-reducing activities, including adherence to medical regimen, staying in treatment, and altering one's habits and activities [KASL, 1975].

Overall, these influences and formulations from psychology and sociology have not only enlarged our understanding of the impact of changes in health status on behavior, and of the possible motivating forces behind behaviors which have health consequences. They have also served as a useful reminder that not all mediating processes between the environment and some illness outcome need be via altered biological processes, but can be also via altered behavior and functioning with their own consequent health status changes. This reminder has been just as useful for social epidemiology as for psychosomatic medicine. (We shall have occasion to return to this point in discussing several of the chapters in this volume, particularly the one on migration.)

There is one area of studies which probably best exemplifies the common interests of social epidemiology and psychosomatic medicine: the area generally labelled 'social stress and disease'. A quick examination of the literature dealing with conceptualization and definition of stress [APPLEY and TRUMBULL, 1967; BONNER, 1967; ENGEL, 1962; GROEN and BASTIAANS, 1975; LAZARUS, 1966, 1971; LIPOWSKI, 1975; MCGRATH, 1970; RUFF and KORCHIN, 1967; SELLS, 1970; WEITZ, 1970] leads to the conclusion that the term 'stress' has not achieved any kind of a closure, either in the sense of concept clarification or as delineation of boundaries. Given this lack of convergence, it would seem that the best way to treat the concept of 'stress' is as a pretheoretical term (i.e., as taken over from the vernacular and prior to any conceptual refinement) with an open-ended definition which consists of enumeration of environmental conditions which are to be considered stressful. Such enumerations may be either in terms of concrete instances (e.g., death of spouse) or in terms of more abstract, theoretical terminology (e.g., information overload). Since stress formulations are usually tied to a particular field of study and cannot be easily extended to all levels of human functioning [SCOTT and HOWARD, 1970], it will probably be necessary to enumerate stresses separately for different settings, such as the work setting [e.g., GROSS, 1970; LANDY and TRUMBO, 1976; MCGRATH, 1976].

The form of 'social stress' which recent studies both in social epidemiology and psychosomatic medicine have found worth their closest attention are *social change* and *life events*. This is probably because events of social change are most likely to encompass one or more of the major meanings of stress: threat, uncertainty and unpredictability, conflict, excessive demands, failure of aspirations, frustration of needs, loss. Investigators, such as CASSEL [1974a], GROEN [1971], HINKLE [1974], HOLMES and MASUDA [1974], KAGAN [1971], and RAHE [1974] have all assigned great significance to social change in the etiology of illness.

There would seem to be two outstanding characteristics of the body of recent studies on social change and illness: (1) the work is largely atheoretical, at least in the sense that the component characteristics of change and the process of reaction-adaptation are seldom explicated, and (2) the studies are usually 1 of 2 kinds: those using some variation of the Schedule of Recent Experience (SRE) instrument, and those examining more intensively one event or social change at a time.

The unsettled theoretical issues in the study of health effects of social change are so fundamental that we have yet to explore even the question: Under what circumstances may 'no change' be expected to have health status consequences which are comparable to the observed effects of some social changes? It has been suggested [GRAHAM, 1974; NEUGARTEN and DATAN, 1974] that, from the life cycle perspective, certain events or changes are 'normative': expected, planned, and desired. When such normal transitions do not take place (or they happen 'too early' or 'too late'), this may create as many adaptive demands on the individual as do many of the social changes which have been studied. The 'person-environment fit' perspective [FRENCH, 1974; FRENCH *et al.*, 1974; VAN HARRISON, in press] leads to a similar concern with 'no change' as the life cycle perspective: if stress is seen as a lack of fit between person characteristics (needs, skills, abilities) and environmental characteristics (demands, resources, supplies), then a significant change in the personal characteristics may create stress if no appropriate, corresponding changes in the environment ('life events') have taken place. Or, alternately, how strong can be the adaptive demands of a life event or change which serves to reduce the existing misfit between the person and his environment?

The basic point, however, is not which life situations of 'no change' should be studied in addition to the social changes already being studied (this might easily degenerate into the simplistic question: what 'no events' should we add to the list of events on the SRE?) but how to build up a theoretical framework which will be sufficiently broad so that one can represent the relationship between the characteristics of the host and of the environment, whether or not one or the other (or both) are changing. This is a tall order, of course, and most of the suggestions which have been offered deal only with assessing some additional characteristics of the change experience.

BROWN [1974] has argued forcefully that we must known the 'context' of an event (i.e., the meaning of the event vis-à-vis the person's plans, aspirations, and goals); however, this suggestion is difficult to implement and propels the investigator into an excessively idiographic, subjectivistic approach, which makes the development of a general theory and a general methodology an unlikely prospect. Subclassifications of life events into 'desirable' and 'undesirable', or 'exits' and 'entrances' [e.g., PAYKEL, 1974] are surely ad hoc, temporizing solutions unlikely to provide major insights. Others have made more systematic suggestions. DOHRENWEND [1977], for example, calls for measuring: the role of the individual in the event, extent of individual's anticipation of the event, extent of control over the occurrence of event, individual's previous experience that is relevant to the event, and social support available to the individual. RABKIN and STRUENING [1976] talk about magnitude (generally the only dimension measured), duration, unpredictability, and novelty. These are useful suggestions but they are not easy to operationalize; moreover, each one carries a potential for both objective and subjective measurement along multiple subdimensions.

Other writers have emphasized the importance of characteristics of the individuals experiencing the change and the social setting in which it takes place. CASSEL [1974], for example, focuses on the greater suceptibility of individuals in subordinate positions (a generalization from both animal and human studies) and on the importance of social buffers and group support.

RAHE [1974] lists certain categories of variables which may be thought of as influencing the causal pathway from stress (social change and life events) to illness: past experience, psychological defences, physiological reaction, coping, and illness behavior. This list, of course, is a useful reminder of the possible complexity of effects, but is no more than a first small step in constructing a skeleton of the requisite theory.

The implementation of all the above suggestions would still not tell us the specifics of a particular change. Consider, for example, the study of promotion. The above suggestions would lead us to find out for each person: (a) the 'context' of the promotion: desired, planned, 'on time' (in the life cycle sense); (b) it is anticipated, the individual had a good deal of influence over it, he has had previous experience with promotions, and social support is high, and (c) the event is 'desirable', appears to be both an 'exit' and an 'entrance', and its duration is uncertain. Yet we would still not known anything about changes in job demands, new skills to be learned, new people to deal with, and so on. Being promoted to a full professor at a major university or to a vice president at a large company may be highly similar events along all the change dimensions; yet, for the former the change in the work environment may be minimal (e.g., less teaching) while for the latter the changes in job demands (e.g., role conflict and role ambiguity, overload) may be major. Should these environmental aspects be ignored?

A similar argument can be built up for other social changes, such as residential moves [KASL, 1972, 1976]. Residential changes may be characterized along all the dimensions suggested for general study of social change and life events, yet unless we also study the specifics of this particular change, we may totally fail in being able to assess its health effects. In addition to specific and definable changes in various physical aspects of the residential environment, residential changes may also involve: (a) segregation from friends and relatives, which may involve reduced social contacts and reduced mutual help and support; (b) unfamiliar surroundings and unknown requirements; (c) new schools, changes in police protection, and so on. Failure to disentangle the possible health benefits due to improvement in physical aspects of housing from the possible adverse effects of the social uprooting has led to inconclusive findings regarding health effects of residential moves. Similarly, the literature on morbidity and mortality effects of involuntary residential moves of institutionalized elderly is quite inconsistent, unless one pays attention to the detailed characteristics of such moves, in particular the extent of social casework provided in order to minimize fear of unknown, to preserve established social relationships, and retain familiar belongings [Kasl, 1972, 1977].

In short, the requisite theoretical framework for the study of health effects of social change must dimensionalize not only the experiential aspects of the change, but also the social-environmental aspects: job change studies need to describe the occupational environments, residential change studies must assess the residential environments, conjugal bereavement studies must examine the (former) marital relationship, and so on. The study of change, in my opinion, must more firmly embrace the ecological perspective of social epidemiology. However, it is also true that those environmentally-oriented investigators who have studied change by simply characterizing and dimensionalizing the before-after environmental difference need to broaden their approach and assess also some of the experiential aspects of the change: degree of anticipation, preparation, previous experience, and so on.

The greater emphasis on the environment in the study of change should also help resolve the issue of boundary between change and no change. The 'no change' for an adolescent who does not go to college can be described in terms of increased social isolation from previous friends who are now away in college. The 'no change' of a woman who remains single can be described in terms of changed associations with same-sex age peers who have all married. The 'no change' of an elderly woman who has lived at the same address for 40 years can be described in terms of the increased frequency of violent attacks on the elderly by young hoodlums, which are taking place on her street.

Given these comments above, it is difficult for me to see how the dominant methodology in the study of health effects of social change, the use of the SRE (or a similar instrument) together with some scaling procedure to arrive at a total score, can significantly advance our present knowledge. This methodology has been extensively reviewed, evaluated, and criticized [e.g., Birley and Connolly, 1976; Dohrenwend and Dohrenwend, 1974; Rabkin and Struening, 1976], and the criticism appears thoughtful and justified. The salient criticism can be summarized along the following lines: (1) The set of weights used for assigning scores to events may be inappropriate or nonoptimal, given cultural, subcultural, and individual differences in rating such events. (2) Aside from magnitude, other characteristics of each event should also be known: previous experience with event, anticipation and preparation for it, duration, desirability, person's role in the event, etc. (3) Many of the so-called events are vague with no specific objective referrents. (4) There may be conceptual and methodological overlap between the independent variable (life 'events') and the dependent variable (health status indicator). (5) Biases in recalling and reporting events may produce spurious association between life events and health status (particularly so in retrospective studies). (6) Onset of many events and many health status changes is difficult to determine, making it impossible to establish temporal order, so crucial to causal interpretations. (7) Illness behavior is often confused with illness. (8) The global (total) score precludes a meaningful study of conditioning variables (in the person and in the environment) and of intervening processes.

This list of criticisms is familiar, rather than innovative or definitive. With accumulating evidence it is likely to grow rather than shrink. Some points are relatively unimportant (e.g., the use of different sets of weights still generally lead to highly correlated total scores) while others are crucial (e.g., biases and confounding, causal interpretation). And, of course, the list of solutions is quite short, with some of these not being all that helpful. For example, prospective studies are not necessarily the panacea they are claimed to be. Thus, if there are individuals who characteristically over-report both events (particularly the vague ones) and symptoms, then the measurement of events at one point in time and of symptoms at a later point in no way removes this bias. A more adequate data analysis, such as cross-lagged correlations [COOK and CAMPBELL, 1976], might provide a better handle on this problem.

The cumulative effects of this criticism should be seriously examined and may even call for a moratorium on SRE-type research. However, such a call [WERSHOW and REINHART, 1974] was promptly rejected [CAPLAN, 1975]. Why should this be? I believe there may be 2 reasons for this: (1) The SRE and related instruments have given rise to a large and growing body of research which deals with issues which are not substantive in the original sense (i.e., change and illness) but are either concerned with new issues of substance (e.g., sociocultural influences on perception and evaluation of certain symbolic stimuli, words and phrases describing 'life events') and with methodological issues (e.g., reliability and validity, memory, systematic biases, approaches to scaling). This research is apparently seen as worthwhile in its own right and not in need of any 'external' justification, such as how it leads to an improved methodology in the study of health effects of change. (2) Historians of science tell us that only clearly formulated theories with unambiguous deductions are vulnerable to disconfirmation and thus can be clearly rejected. Vague theories are not vulnerable to new empirical evidence, but instead get revised and become more complex; only a better theory leads to their gradual disappearance. Perhaps the same is true of research instruments. The SRE-type methodology usually produces 'positive' results, even though such findings are likely to be ambiguous and compatible with several interpretations. But unless someone offers a better methodology, this convenient instrument will continue being used, even though it may call for increasingly lengthy and complex disclaimers and reservations.

MECHANIC [1974, p. 87], in his thoughtful overview of the literature on stressful life events, concludes: 'It is clear that stressful life events play some role in the occurrence of illness in populations. But any statement beyond this vague generalization is likely to stir controversy. The important issues in understanding how life events interact with social psychological, biological, and intrapsychic variables require specification of *what events* influence *what* illnesses under *what* conditions through *what* processes?'

This conclusion – that one must examine intensively one social event at a time if we are to advance beyond vague generalizations – seems almost inevitable in light of the foregoing discussion and criticisms. We must not forget that most such 'life events' are so firmly embedded in a large network of prior events, decisions, reactions, and copings, that the investigator's assumption that he is dealing with a before-after design, with the events anchored solidly in time in between, is all too often a radiant illusion. The study of life events, after all, is a study of lifes in progress.

The suggestion, then, is that adavances in our knowledge are more likely to take place if we study intensively single events (and the surrounding other changes thereby precipitated) than if we wait for the crucial methodological improvements in the SRE-type approach. However, this siggestion is hardly enough to guarantee progress. We also need research designs which will permit causal inferences and in which the role of confounding variables is brought under at least partial control. For example, the study of single events, such as voluntary residential moves to the suburbs, have failed to demonstrate any consequences of the moves which could not be interpreted as 'intended' changes, i.e., the reasons for which the move was made in the first place – increased satisfaction with housing, increased social life, and so on [KASL, 1976]. In other words, such residential moves are so firmly embedded in life cycle variables, in goals, aspirations, plans, intentions, and perceived opportunities, that unidirectional causal inferences, located in time, are nearly impossible. Stated another way, certain events and certain settings permit more effective research designs than others. Consider, for example, the contrast between studying the mental and physical health effects of bereavement vs. dissolution of marriage. It is easy to see that the former can be (on the average) a much more discrete event with a discernible onset and with fewer confounding variables, enmeshing both the independent and dependent variables.

It would appear that in the study of social change we must be dilligently on the lookout for research opportunities represented by the 'natural experiment'. By this term I mean those planned and/or predictable events, such as urban renewal or automation of a plant, which: (a) are socially significant; (b) are believed to be stressful (in the sense that they are likely to have consequences for the mental and physical health of the people involved); (c) can contribute to our basic knowledge about stress effects and adaptation, and (d) which can tell us something about managing such changes with a minimum of destructive impact. These events can be studied in their natural setting, frequently with a good deal of scientific rigor. When the individual's exposure to such events takes place with a minimum of self-selection and when adequate comparison groups, not exposed to such events, can be found, then we have a truly adequate compromise between naturalistic observations and laboratory experimental manipulation. Incidentally, while these comments concern the study of 'stressful events', they are equally applicable to socially planned interventions which are intended to be of benefit to some target individuals [CAMPBELL, 1969]; there is a growing methodological literature designed to help the investigator working with quasi-experimental designs in the field setting [e.g., ABERT and KAMRASS, 1974; BENNETT and LUMSDAINE, 1975; CAPORASO and ROOS, 1973; COOK and CAMPBELL, 1976; KENNY, 1975; STANLEY, 1967].

The comments in this section were intended to introduce the reader to the broad perspective (biases?) from which I shall be discussing the various contributions to this volume, and to sensitize him to some of the important issues. Essentially, it seems to me almost axiomatic that when we are working in the domain of social factors (or, more narrowly, stress or change) in health-illness, the etiological picture is bound to be a very complex one. Consequently, we need to be more thoughtful about the problem of selecting an adequately powerful research setting/design. In addition to this general point, it is well to be concerned with one or more of the following issues: (1) Distinguish between the physical and the social environment, and identify and measure relevant aspects of both. (2) Distinguish between the objective events (or objective environment) and subjective perceptions or evaluations of these; determine when it is important to know the relationship between these two; and establish the implications of studying only one or the other. (3) Be on the lookout for different temporal patterns of physiological variables or of health effects, such as proximal vs. distal outcomes, their sequence or their interaction. (4) Consider the relevance of coping behaviors and behavioral adaptations (and other intervening processes) which may modify strikingly the outcome variable. (5) Determine which subgroups (whether defined sociodemographically, by situational variables, or by stable personal characteristics) might be most vulnerable to the effects of the social factor under study.

Commentary on Contributions to this Volume

Coronary Heart Disease
C. DAVID JENKINS

The chapter on coronary heart disease (CHD) is an excellent illustration of the growing overlap between the disciplines of social epidemiology and psychosomatic medicine, since both disciplines have had a long-standing interest in the disease. Moreover, certain problems which plague us in the study of other diseases and conditions are less obtrusive in the case of CHD, thus permitting us a clearer view of the substantive issues involved in the psychosocial etiology of CHD. For example, the role of several biological risk factors is reasonably well understood [for a recent review see KULLER, 1976] and their contributions have been quantified in multiple logistic risk-factor equations, thus allowing us more easily to assess the independent or interactive contribution of a particular psychosocial variable. Secondly, problems of classification-diagnosis are not severe, thus giving us a resonable assurance that the same condition is being assessed in different studies. However, it is becoming increasingly obvious [JENKINS, 1976] that one needs to keep track separately of myocardial infarction (MI) and angina pectoris (AP) since the two are likely to involve a different set of psychosocial risk factors. Moreover, the classification of AP is based on 'softer' data and we are beginning to understand some of the biases which might be involved in perceiving and/or reporting clinical symptoms of coronary disease [e.g., CROOG and LEVINE, 1969; REEDER *et al.*, 1973]. The methodological significance of these studies would presumably apply to the classification of 'silent' MI, as well. Thirdly, narrow etiological formulations involving a single psychosocial factor or a single constellation of factors (e.g., specific conflict) appear to be past history for both psychosocial epidemiology and psychosomatic medicine (for an exception, see GROEN [1976], who postulates that 3 factors – lack of occupational success, a certain family situation, and an inability to cope with or compensate for the failure – have to co-occur if CHD is to develop), and a more pragmatic, richer exploration of many possible psychosocial factors is characteristic of current studies.

The JENKINS chapter (which ideally should be read in conjunction with his 1971 and 1976 *New Engl. J. Med.* reviews) is a masterful organization of a diverse, scattered literature which resists easy summary and integration (see ORTH-GOMER [1974] for another attempt to provide framework and structure to this whole literature). With JENKINS' help, the reader can see the major classes of variables studied and can readily conclude which areas are yielding cumulative, convergent evidence, as opposed to evidence which is increasingly more confusing, inconsistent, and divergent.

Global sociological indicators are easily studied variables which have remained opaque as CHD risk factors. For example, marital status is related to CHD mortality; however, so is mortality for every other major cause [National Center for Health Statistics, 1970]. Moreover, while marital status does not seem to exert its causal influence via the traditional cardiovascular risk factors, the path of influence remains unknown. Some 20 years ago, a number of writers [e.g., CHEN and COBB, 1960; KRAUS and LILIENFELD, 1959; LAHORGUE, 1960] proposed several plausible interpretations for the association of marital status with morbidity and mortality, and we are no closer in being able to pin down the most appropriate one now than we were then. Similar comments apply to the association between low educational status and CHD mortality, except that one of the risk factors, blood pressure, does bear some association with educational status [National Center for Health Statistics, 1966], and smoking may as well [STERLING and WEINKMAN, 1976].

Differences in CHD rates across specific occupations remain a promising area of investigation, even as it has become clear that an overall linear gradient in CHD rates with social class or occupational status does not exist in contemporary US. For example, analysis of mortality due to arteriosclerotic heart disease among US withe males aged 20–64, by occupations [GURALNICK, 1963], leads to the observation that certain occupational groups (e.g., college presidents – professors – instructors; teachers) have rates lower than expected while other groups (e.g., lawyers and judges; physicians and surgeons; pharmacists; insurance agents and brokers; real estate agents and brokers) have considerably higher rates than expected. Since these differences are reasonably large (about two to one), but involve groups rather comparable on social status, level of physical activity, physical hazards in the work environment, and so on, it is not unreasonable to ask whether differences in specific job demands and job-related activities might not be involved in the etiological picture. Of course, the effective study of 'stress' at work is not an easy matter (COOPER and MARSHALL [1976] and KASL [in press] review this literature in some detail), but we can certainly go beyond the primitive research design utilized by RUSSEK [1962] and similar later studies [e.g., FRIEDMAN and HELBERSTEIN, 1968].

Religious affiliation and religious attendance continue to be studied in relation to CHD [JENKINS, 1976], but failure to replicate previously observed differences seems to be a common fate of initially promising results. At this point, the best guess would seem to be that unless one is studying religious groups with known and striking differences in life styles and habits (such as Mormons and Seventh Day Adventists), CHD differences due to religion are likely to remain inscrutable and vulnerable to nonreplication.

The work on social mobility and status incongruity appeared initially promising [JENKINS, 1971], but results of more recent studies [JENKINS, 1976] have produced a confusing array of nonreplication and methodological controversy. (Because of the overlap with the chapters on Migration and Occupational Mobility, additional comments on these studies will be offered later.) A pessimistic conclusion from these inconsistent findings would be that they have failed to coalesce into any kind of an interpretable picture and thus cannot help us understand the possible role of social mobility and status incongruity in the psychosocial etiology of CHD. An optimistic conclusion would be that these results point to a good deal of specificity of effects and that the effect of mobility and incongruity will eventually form a coherent and consistent picture once the other relevant variables, with which they apparently interact, are considered at the same time. Stated somewhat differently, this would imply that mobility and incongruity are 'phenotypic', surrogate variables which are linked to different 'genotypic' variables, depending on various additional characteristics of the study population. Thus we may see a replication of the KAPLAN *et al.* [1971] results of opposite CHD correlates of mobility in upper- and middle-class vs. lower-class subjects in future studies – provided social class is the crucial variable for revealing the 'latent structure' of the mobility dimension. In fact, WARDWELL *et al.* [1968] did show that CHD rates were more adversely affected by intergenerational mobility of lower social class men than of middle or upper class men; however, they also obtained complex interactions with religious status which cry out for replication.

WARDWELL and BAHNSON's failure to replicate the CHD correlates of cultural mobility in Southeastern Connecticut, which SYME originally observed in North Dakota and California, may still be reconciled with a well-reasoned argument showing that cultural mobility has a different meaning depending on whether the subjects live in more recently settled, more agricultural regions of the US vs. in older, more urban parts of the country. Similarly, the findings of MEDALIE's study of Israeli government employees that MI rates were higher among first generation Israeli than among immigrants appear to contradict the simple notion that it is the immigrant group which is experiencing greatest cultural change and should have highest rates. However, the vast majority of work on acculturation processes has suggested that cultural conflict is greatest in the first generation of new citizens rather than the immigrants themselves and thus the MEDALIE data may not be 'inconsistent'. What this all says, of course, is that complex variables and processes are being related to CHD in a relatively simplistic way, and that a good deal of conceptual and methodological explication of these variables is needed if we are to move beyond keeping a simple tally of how many studies do and do not support some general association. (The later chapters on Migration and Occupational Mobility will provide an opportunity to make this observation in greater depth.)

The WILLIAMS' findings of higher CHD rates among the Western Collaborative Group Study men who had *fewer* job changes are particularly disconcerting in view of an earlier finding [JENKINS *et al.*, 1966] from the same population: men with 'silent' myocardial infarction were more likely to have received a job promotion within the previous 3 years than age-occupation matched controls. And since LEHMAN *et al.* [1967] found no association between many indices of occupational mobility and CHD mortality, we again have the situation of results all over the place and a need for a more probing, refined use of the independent variable.

Status incongruity continues being explored as a possible risk factor for CHD [JENKINS, 1976] and one again has the impression that the results are quite fragile. Moreover, there is a good deal of methodological controversy regarding the adequacy of data analysis in the status incongruity studies, particularly the extent to which main effects (due to individual status dimensions such as education or occupational level) have been removed before one searches for interaction (incongruity) [see HORAN and GRAY, 1974; SHEKELLE, 1976]. The particular incongruity which may be most promising as a risk factor is the combination of relatively low education with relatively high occupational level in men [BRUHN *et al.*, 1968; CHRISTENSON and HINKLE, 1961; HINKLE *et al.,* 1966, 1968; WAN, 1971]. Conceptually, this might represent a work situation in which the job demands exceed the skills and training of the man, leading to work pressures and overload. This in turn would permit linking this form of incongruity with the suggestive literature on work pressures and CHD [e.g., HOUSE, 1974; JENKINS, 1971; ZOHMAN, 1973]. However, this interpretation of this form of status incongruity must be applied cautiously: HINKLE and his collaborators have clearly shown that the men without college education who go on to attain high occupational status in the Bell system are different from the college-educated men on so many diverse variables (smoking, social background, non-work activities) that the college-no college distinction picks up broad differences in early established life styles rather than just the narrow congruity-incongruity distinction.

The literature which JENKINS summarizes under the heading of 'anxiety and neuroticism' [see also JENKINS, 1971, 1976] is in sufficient agreement regarding the fact that persons with AP or MI are likely to be higher on various indices of poor mental health, so that further retrospective, case-control studies of this kind are quite unnecessary – unless, of course, one is studying the mental health consequences of having CHD and one has some new hypothesis about how patients cope with or respond to the illness. No on has ever convincingly proposed a control group of patients with another disease which would so adequately control for effects of having CHD that any differences in anxiety-neuroticism which obtained between CHD patients and controls could then be interpreted as having etiological significance for CHD. Moreover, most symptom-based indices of psychopathology are developed for use on physically healthy subjects and their validity is thrown in doubt when applied to patients with physical illnesses.

The evidence from prospective studies would seem to suggest that many aspects of 'neuroticism' may indeed be antecedent to AP, but not MI. What may be predictive of MI is perhaps a much narrower set of variables dealing with slepp disturbances, tiredness at the beginning or the end of a day, and not being able to relax. JENKINS' discussion of these findings, however, makes it clear that even this generalization must be a tentative one since many of the prospective studies are simply longitudinal follow-ups of an unselected sample of subjects rather than a selection of an initially healthy cohort. Since MI is a risk factor for another MI, since AP is a risk factor for MI (particularly in men), since subclinical disease progresses on to clinical manifestations – and since all of these can influence the above set of 'predictors' – the causal pathways are not clear unless one starts out with a demonstrably healthy cohort.

The studies dealing with 'life dissatisfactions' are not easily separable from the above studies of 'anxiety-neuroticism', since we are inevitably dealing with correlated variables. (Possibly one difference is that while higher anxiety and mental distress are consequences of CHD which our intuition readily accepts, changes in life satisfaction as a consequence of CHD are perhaps less intuitively compelling without some evidence.) And it is thus not surprising that the evidence for life dissatisfaction as a risk factor is suggestive for AP but not very promising for MI. However, a recent report [THEORELL and FLODERUS-MYRHED, 1977] does suggest that one area of life dissatisfaction, the work role, may be related prospectively to MI, while another area, the family, clearly is not. Various other studies have zeroed in on job dissatisfaction and complaints about work in relation to CHD or CHD risk factors [e.g., GROEN and DRORY, 1967; HOUSE, 1972; MEDALIE *et al.*, 1973; SALES and HOUSE, 1971; THEORELL and RAHE, 1972], using a variety of methodologies and approaches. These studies (almost exclusively of men) do support the notion that the work role is the most promising area for more intensive scrutiny; but the growing list of studies finding no association with job dissatisfaction must not be ignored [e.g., CAPLAN, 1971; CAPLAN *et al.*, 1975; MUELLER, 1965; SCHÄR *et al.*, 1973; WARDWELL and BAHNSON, 1973].

Studies of 'coronary-prone behavior pattern' (type A) are concerned with perhaps the most promising and most busily researched psychosocial risk factor in the whole CHD area. The measurement of this pattern is quite varied, including the Friedman-Rosenman interview, the Jenkins Activity Survey, and various ad hoc modifications, abbreviations, and innovations. Overall, the following conclusions appear justified: (1) type A behavior is a prospectively established risk factor for CHD (among men) and the increased risk is independent of other firmly established risk factors [ROSENMAN *et al.*, 1975; BRAND *et al.*, 1976]. (2) Among men with a single previous CHD event, type A behavior increases the risk for reoccurrence of CHD, independent of other risk factors [JENKINS *et al.*, 1976]. (3) The dichotomous, clinical judgment of Friedman-Rosenman predicts CHD better than a self-report measure, the Jenkins Activity Scale [JENKINS *et al.*, 1974]; the loss in predictive power is about what one would expect from calculating the error of misclassification [MACMAHON and PUGH, 1970] due to using the self-report test instead of the clinical judgment (see JENKINS *et al.*

[1971] for the association between the 2 measures). (4) Factor analysis of the self-report test has yielded three factors (hard-driving, job involvement, and speed and impatience), but there are many other items which do not load on any of these three factors [ZYZANSKI and JENKINS, 1970]. Moreover, the three factors are useless in predicting new CHD or recurrence [JENKINS *et al.,* 1974, 1976], since only the total scale score predicts. On the job involvement factor, men who go on to develop CHD are, against expectation, slightly (nonsignificantly) lower than men who remain healthy.

The most striking characteristic of the work on type A is that even though this dimension of behavior is conceptualized as the result of a predisposition stimulated by appropriate environmental challenges (as FRIEDMAN and ROSENMAN [1974] state, '...an environmental challenge must always serve as the fuse for this...' behavior pattern), the actual studies mostly treat it as a stable personality characteristic which by itself is an adequate predictor of CHD, no matter what the environmental setting. As a minimum, we need some information about the occupational specificity-generality of type A behavior as a risk factor; the basic work derives from a fairly limited set of occupations (middle- and upper-level managerial and technical-scientific positions). Ideally, we need to break down this risk factor into 3 components: (a) the relevant personality predisposition; (b) the demands of a particular (work) setting, and (c) the behavior and reaction which are precipitated when these demands 'activate' the predisposition.

A second characteristic of the work with type A behavior is that this complex concept has resisted conceptual and methodological clarification and purification. The 3 factors obtained by ZYZANSKI and JENKINS [1970] appear to have surprisingly little practical utility and account for a smallish amount of the total variance; in other words, the 3 factors alone clearly do not add up to the total concept. On the other hand, the global, dichotomous clinical judgment of Friedman-Rosenman has remained a black box which presumably hides answers to many traditional psychometric questions pertaining to combinatorial clinical ratings: (a) on what information in the interview or elsewhere are various component ratings based; (b) how are the components combined (using what implicit set of weights); (c) are some components better predictors of CHD than other components, and (d) what is the relative importance of subject's self-report vs. observer's ratings as sources of data.

Several studies cited by JENKINS [1976] would seem to suggest that impatient overactivity, and excessive competitiveness and job involvement without a sense of accomplishment, joy, or relief (the 'Sisyphus reaction') may be the crucial components of type A behavior, while others, such as aggressivity, may eventually drop out. Other questions concerning possible refinements of the concept can be raised: Can one adequately separate the 'Sisyphus reaction' from equally high levels of job involvement and activity carried out with a sense of mastery, challenge and joy (avoidance vs. approach work motivation; tension-exhaustion vs. 'thriving' on pressure)? Are certain behaviors of 'speed and impatience' merely characteristic of individual life-style habits, while others are in response to stress and tension, and does this distinction have any significance for CHD risk?

The recent work of GLASS and collaborators [e.g., GLASS *et al.*, 1974] has begun to explicate the type A dimension in terms of other concepts, such as the need to have control over various aspects of one's environment and the resultant reactions of helplessness-tension-hyperactivity when such control appears impossible. However, it is difficult to evaluate the promise of this direction, since such studies are conducted on young adults and without any health-related outcomes.

The complexity of the concept of type A behavior is also reflected in the inconclusiveness of results from studies which have examined specific aspects of the work setting most likely to 'arouse' type A behavior. For example, working excessive hours and/or holding down more than one full-time job appears to be associated with CHD morbidity and mortality, especially among younger men. But it is not clear what exactly is involved. THEORELL and RAHE [1972] found that cases with CHD had worked more hours overtime, but controls had spent more time doing work at home (i.e., taking their work home). BRUHN *et al.* [1968] found no differences in overtime work, only in having more than one job. And a mortality analysis [BUELL and BRESLOW, 1960] revealed a gradient primarily among younger, light workers, but not among workers doing either sedentary, or medium-to-heavy work (farmers and farm workers were excluded altogether). The literature dealing with job demands and job pressures appears similarly complex or inconclusive. THEORELL and FLODERUS-MYRHED [1977] found that building construction workers, who later developed MI, reported on a 'workload' index an excess of items reflecting both too much and too little responsibility. And in the earlier case-control study [THEORELL and RAHE, 1972], cases with MI reported *fewer* responsibilities at work and *less* supervising of others than did matched controls. Tax accountants have higher cholesterol levels as tax deadline approaches than they do at other times of the year [FRIEDMAN *et al.*, 1958]; however, men responsible for launching the space vehicle for moon landing and working under severe deadline pressure are no different from controls (without any responsibility for the launch) on EKG abnormalities, cholesterol, blood pressure, and glucose [REYNOLDS, 1974]. Air traffic controllers, especially those working in high density traffic areas, may [COBB and ROSE, 1973] or may not CAPLAN *et al.*, 1975] have higher blood pressure levels. In short, it is too early to insist on the generalization that jobs or organizational roles which are associated with overload, excessive demands, and many responsibilities represent settings of high CHD risk [SALES, 1969].

The work on behavior type A is proliferating rapidly and more and more of the recent studies are anchoring this variable in other social-psychological data, including the occupational setting [e.g., METTLIN, 1976; SHEKELLE *et al.*, 1976], instead of studying it as an isolated psychosocial predictor of CHD.

I agree with JENKINS' conclusion that 'the primary research need in this area [psychological risk factors in CHD] is not for further exploratory studies, but rather for carefully designed hypothesis-testing studies which will serve to sort out and clarify the exciting but disorganized array of positive findings' (p. 16). I only wish it were possible to provide the reader with a little more of a detailed blueprint to follow. Essentially, the many contradictory and partially replicated findings suggest that some hypotheses are more promising than others, some measures are more probing than others, some settings are more effective than others. But it is difficult to identify the ones which will most likely advance our understanding and build on existing knowledge. Given this uncertainty, it is a good bet that the next generation of studies will simply have to be more complex (at least in the sense of number of variables assessed and analyzed) and more concerned with the specifics of *interaction* among the variables which have shown some association with CHD. The major classes of interacting variables are: (a) the traditional biological risk factors; (b) the behavioral risk factors (e.g., smoking, diet); (c) the social ecological variables (social change, work setting, social support); (d) the personality dimensions and psychological reactions (e.g., anxiety-tension, vulnerability to exhaustion and the 'Sisyphus reaction', predisposition to type A behaviors), and (e) the sociodemographic and background factors.

Sociocultural Change and Blood Pressure
A.M. OSTFELD and D.A. D'ATRI

This chapter zeroes in on a specific segment of the work on psychosocial epidemiology of high blood pressure (for other recent reviews dealing with different segments of this work, see BENSON and GUTMAN [1974]; MUSTACCHI [1976], STAHL *et al.* [1975]; a good deal of the international data on blood pressure is contained in the WHO volume [HATANO *et al.,* 1976]: cross-cultural differences in blood pressure distributions (mean, association with age) which might be attributable to differences in certain societal characteristics reflecting the dimension from stable and traditional to changing , nontraditional, westernized. The methodology of the studies reviewed is mostly a mixture of medical anthropology and descriptive epidemiology.

Since OSTFELD and D'ATRI do such a convincing job of demolishing the methodological and substantive credibility of the presumed evidence, it may be difficult for the reader to recapture the original excitment and promise of the hypothesis that living in stable, traditional societies is associated with lower blood pressure levels which do not rise with age. Essentially, it had been part of accepted medical wisdom that (a) rise in blood pressure is part of 'normal' aging and (b) blood pressure levels may be a sensitive indicant of 'stress' in many individuals. The observation that there may be societies around the world in which blood pressure levels do not rise with age seemed to have a dual impact: (a) it held promise for a more objective study of cross-cultural differences in stress in relation to societal structure, and (b) it suggested that increased blood pressure with age was not a universal biological norm but could perhaps be interpreted as the accumulated impact of living in more stressful societies and settings.

It is characteristic of the process of dissemination of scientific ideas and knowledge that socially significant hypotheses (especially the more general ones) undergo swings from enthusiastic acceptance to searching, methodological criticism. Scientific progress is served if such acceptance leads to research which would not otherwise be done, and if such criticism leads to the recognition of ways to carry out better executed studies. Progress is not served if such acceptance is short-circuited into dogma, or if such criticism leads to the abandonment of further studies.

JOHN CASSEL was perhaps the foremost proponent of the sociocultural change-high blood pressure hypothesis. A careful reading of his recent brief article [CASSEL, 1974b] reveals that even as he reaffirmed his belief in the fruitfulness of the hypothesis, he also saw the limitations of the previous evidence. Consequently, he zeroed in on the before-after study of both migrants and nonmigrants (e.g., PRIOR's work) as the most precise design with which to investigate the hypothesis of sociocultural change. And he specifically recommended the study of various intervening variables, including dietary ones.

Ostfeld and D'Atri offer the conclusion that the association between rapid sociocultural change and greater prevalence of high blood pressure involves the intermediary mechanism of diet changes and weight gain, and that it is *un*necessary to postulate stressful social processes. (A reference to dietary changes in salt intake as well would make the postulated intermediary mechanism even more comprehensive and defensible.) This conclusion is unassailable if interpreted as a criticism of previous studies for failing to control for the effects of diet changes-weight gain, or as pointing to the absolute necessity of future studies to asses the influence of this parameter. However, since only a few of the numerous studies reviewed permit a *quantitative* documentation that the associated weight gain can account for *all* of the blood pressure differential, this conclusion must be viewed not as a definitive reinterpretation of all of the evidence but as a substitution of a simpler, more plausible, and more easily defended hypothesis. In fact, we do not really know whether a diligent search and reanalysis of existing evidence (perhaps to be carried out in the near future as the interpretive pendulum begins to swing somewhat away from the Ostfeld-D'Atri position) would not reveal some residual contribution of sociocultural change in a few studies. Furthermore, it is possible that social stress interacts, in the long run, with the effects of greater obesity or of greater salt intake. But in a simlpe 2 group study design in wich diet and stress are confounded, it would be difficult to develop an actuarial formula which would detect such an interaction.

It might be noted in passing that there is very little documentation of the statistical reliability of the purported difference in slope of blood pressure on age, between stable and changing societies. This is somewhat reminiscent of earlier claims of observed bimodalities in distributions of continuous biological parameters such as blood pressure or serum uric acid, since such claims would have supported the preconceived notion that hypertension or hyperuricemia were distinct entities. However, such bimodalities turned out to be merely statistically unreliable irregularities in the tail ends of essentially normal distributions.

Ultimately, the difference between the Cassel and the Ostfeld-D'Atri position is one of scientific strategy in the application of the rule of parsimony in the explanation of a set of findings. It would seem to me that in looking back on past evidence there is some preference for scientific explanations to be parsimonious and involving, whenever possible, simple well-understood mediating processes. This is because more complex explanations, involving poorly understood mediating processes, tend to be less precise, and are thus invulnerable to refutation by empirical evidence – surely an undesirable property. However, when looking forward to future studies, complex and less parsimonious explanations may be preferable if one is dealing with complex phenomena. There is some danger that parsimonious explanations used as hypotheses to be tested in future studies may prevent the richness of thinking that should go into designing a study, collecting data on a multiplicity of variables, and analyzing the findings.

Consider, for example, the study design in which the hypothesis regarding rapid sociocultural change is examined not just by contrasting 2 groups and assessing their blood pressure, dietary habits, and weight, but in which one also assesses in individuals living in the 'modern' or urban setting the extent to which they have held on to their 'traditional' or rural practices. Now we have a possibility for disentangling the two hypotheses: those who retain the traditional ways in the modern setting are more likely to be comparable on dietary practices to those living in the stable, traditional society (or, minimally, they should certainly not be different in diet from all others in the modern setting), but they are likely to experience the greatest amount of sociocultural conflict (stress?). The results reported by SCOTCH [1963] revealed that Zulus living in urban settings had higher blood pressures if they maintained traditional cultural practices – a finding compatible with the sociocultural change hypothesis. However, the recent data on Japanese-Americans [MARMOT and SYME, 1976] showed that those who had retained a traditional Japanese culture had the lowest prevalence of coronary heart disease – a finding compatible with the dietary hypothesis, though not necessarily completely accounted for by it.

In the above example it was assumed that retention of traditional ways while living in a modern, nontraditional setting heightens the conflict and the presumed stress effects. But why should not it have the opposite effect: buffer the individual against experiencing the change too rapidly? Perhaps it does, but only if the individual can find others who similarly maintain traditional ways (a residential enclave, or perhaps only a social network of relatives and friends). Well, the point of these speculations is not to settle anything in the armchair, but only to reveal the potential complexity of the underlying processes – which is in stark contrast to the inchoate simplicity with which the sociocultural hypothesis is stated and tested in most of the studies reviewed by OSTFELD and D'ATRI.

Ultimately, we must look to the migration studies for both richer theoretical formulations and more probing research designs (i.e., longitudinal studies). Therefore, I shall return to some of these issues in the discussion of PRIOR's chapter.

Anorexia Nervosa
A.H. CRISP and O.W. HILL

The reader who wishes to gain a general overview of the topic of anorexia nervosa (AN) need not consult very many publications: the present two chapters by CRISP and HILL (plus some of their related publications, e.g., Crisp [1970] and HILL [1976a]), the 1972 volume in this series of Advances [REICHSMAN, 1972], and perhaps the two chapters in the *American Handbook of Psychiatry* [BRUCH, 1974, 1975]. A perusal of these publications leads to the quick realization that: (a) our knowledge about AN is based on cases in treatment, and (b) there are no epidemiological studies of AN in the population (though there are some surveys of relevant symptoms and experiences, such as dieting behavior, weight losses of specifiied magnitude, secondary amenorrhea, etc.).

CRISP and HILL are acknowledged experts on AN, with rich clinical and investigative experience, and they do a fine job of summarizing the evidence in a way which permits the reader to understand its limitations and see the real obstacles to carrying out a convincing epidemiological study of AN. Some of the evidence seems beyond reasonable doubt: the preponderance of females, the typical onset in adolescence, and the high frequency of dieting to achieve weight loss in the developmental sequence of AN. Other evidence is less convincing and is bound up with the problem of studying only cases in treatment and with the adequacy of case-control comparisons: higher social class of cases of AN, premorbid obesity, birth order in relation to unaffected sibs, psychiatric illness in other family members. The general data on 'the social psychology of dieting' [DWYER *et al.*, 1970] are helpful only in suggesting why the attack rate is greatest among adolescent females, but does nothing to explain why the dieting behavior took such a pathological turn. Expert opinion is particularly divergent regarding the extent to which the metabolic and hormonal abnormalities and other somatic manifestations should be considered secondary consequences of starvation. There are also behavioral and attitudinal accompaniments of AN – extreme fear of weight gain, denial of dangers to one's health, distortions of body image, and so on – which again may be either of etiological significance or they may be secondary to the development of AN, a way of responding to and resisting the extreme social pressures to change and start eating normally again.

CASSEL [1974] has suggested that the contribution of epidemiology to the study of psychiatric conditions can be primarily in the resolution of three interrelated problems: (1) identification of cases vs. non-cases; (2) relative utility of theories invoked to explain processes determining the condition being studied, and (3) relative skill with which independent variables are selected as indicators of these determinant processes. These comments are particularly germane to the study of AN.

It would seem that the identification of cases is going to be difficult when: (a) etiology is unknown; (b) it is difficult to distinguish between criterial signs and symptoms vs. secondary clinical manifestations; (c) indicants of severity of condition are easily confused with indicants of security of diagnosis; (d) relevant criteria are assessed with usually 'soft' methodology (e.g., subject's self-observation and reports of past history, interpretive clinical judgements), and (e) relevant criteria are continuous variables and arbitrary cutoff decisions have to be made (e.g., amount of weight loss). This list appears tailor-made for AN and it is not surprising that potential studies of the epidemiology of AN would likely stumble over the most basic issue, case enumeration.

Much can be learned from examinig the developments in the epidemiologic study of other diseases or conditions in which case identification was also a severe initial stumbling block. Rheumatoid arthritis is a good case in point and COBB's book on *The Frequency of Rheumatic Diseases* [1971] offers a good overview of the way a scientific community of involved 'experts' goes about dealing with the problem. The essential steps in this bootstrap operation appear to be as follows. First, the creation of an expert committee on diagnostic criteria. Their function is not to arrive at the truth, but to have enough clout to insist that near-future investigations collect certain types of data in certain ways and apply certain types of rules for diagnostic classification (e.g., absent, possible, probable, definite). Second, broad-based epidemiological surveys in which data on all signs and symptoms of diagnostic significance are reported in such a complete way that all possible interrelationships among them can be examined, different alternate diagnostic rules explored, and the sensitivity/specificity of individual bits of information (or in some combinations) can be computed in relation to them. The National Health Examination Survey of Rheumatoid Arthritis [National Center for Health Statistics, 1966a] is a model study for such a survey and data presentation. Thirdly, after a 'suitable' number of epidemiological studies – both descriptive ones as well as analytical ones dealing with etiological hypotheses – are available for review, the expert committee on diagnostic criteria meets again and evaluates the need for any revisions in criteria.

It is readily apparent that the study of AN has not progressed this far.

HILL cites the Feighner criteria for diagnosis of AN, but appears lukewarm in accepting them. It is also unclear whether there are actually any studies whatever which have applied (or tried to apply) such criteria. Operationalization of these criteria would certainly be difficult; combinatorial rules are not spelled out.

The above statements regarding progress in the classification and epidemiologic study of rheumatoid arthritis are by no means any kind of a blueprint for future studies of AN. A committee of experts on diagnostic criteria might also impose premature orthodoxy which stifles progress. Moreover, AN is considerably rarer than rheumatoid arthritis and there may be little support (scientific, economic) for broad-based population studies, perhaps only for population studies of higher risk subgroups (i.e., adolescent females). But probably the most serious objection to taking this as a blueprint for research on AN is that it neglects a whole different avenue of thinking and study: namely, that AN must be approached from the developmental viewpoint, as the end product of a certain interaction of forces between the person and the socially significant others around her, so that an initially common and socially acceptable behavior, dieting, becomes transformed into pathological, life-threatening behavior with its own powerful set of reinforcers. The behavior of dieting can be viewed not only as a chain of decisions leading to dieting [DWYER *et al.,* 1970] but as a set of outcomes once dieting begins – outcomes which have their own determinants and reinforces. Anorexia nervosa is an extreme outcome in the sense that either (a) the restraining forces in the social environment have failed to stop the behavior at a less extreme form, or (b) other influences have propelled it beyond the less extreme outcomes. Study of only anorexics who come to medical attention (our current source of data) cannot tell us about the dynamics of negotiating or failing to negotiate the various stages in the process. The 'desperate struggle for control, for a sense of identity and effectiveness', which BRUCH [1974] and others talk about, may only be descriptive of the family setting in wich the escalated battle over eating is being fought, but it may or may not help us understand why the conflict managed to escalate that far.

Aside from these brief comments on future research, it might also be noted that we need to pay much more attention to the biological and social-behavioral effects of starvation or semi-starvation. For example, the wartime study of conscientitious objectors subjected to semi-starvation [KEYS *et al.,* 1950] revealed an obsessive preoccupation with food which appears highly similar to that observed among cases of AN. This may suggest that salience of food may not be a predisposing factor for AN but is an outcome. Semi-starvation imposed on subjects for the purposes of research is not a fundable proposition these days, but various research opportunities do occasionally present themselves. Obese subjects on a starvation diet under medical supervision are one possibility; and any differences in sociobiological outcomes between inpatients and outpatients might suggestively point to social (family setting) variables which may modify effects of starvation. Presumably these are the ones crucial to an understanding of the developmental sequences in AN.

Bereavement and Grief
G.L. KLERMAN and J.E. IZEN

Among the topics covered by this volume, health effects of bereavement would appear to be the one which permits the most convincing research designs and thus should yield the most compelling evidence. The detailed, careful review of evidence by KLERMAN and IZEN reveals this expectation to be somewhat naive and not fully justified. Perhaps a more realistic assessment would be: if the study of health effects of bereavement has yielded evidence which still has this many loose ends and ambiguities, then perhaps we should lower our aspirations about how much we can learn in the near future about the health effects of other, more complex indeterminate social events and situations.

KLERMAN and IZEN quite correctly point to LINDEMANN's work as being a seminal influence on subsequent bereavement studies. Consequently, we might note two aspects of his formulation which bear more recognition. One is that the bereaved people he studied had spouses and relatives who died *suddenly,* in a dramatic disaster; no matter what the age of the deceased, in some sense they all died in the 'prime of their lives'. This is certainly not the numerically predominant bereavement experience and it is therefore legitimate to ask to what extent his formulation is appropriate to the study of different bereavement experiences. The second comment deals with LINDEMANN's characterization of normal vs. atypical grief reaction. Logical analysis would seem to suggest that when we are dealing with two alternate, mutually exclusive states, then the criteria which are used to define one state must be also involved in defining the other (mutually exclusive) state. But LINDEMANN's characteristics of normal and atypical grief are 2 sets of non-overlapping criteria. A bereaved person could go through all the stages of normal grief and also exhibit all 5 characteristics of atypical grief reaction! This conceptualization poses severe logical and methodological problems which call for some revisions.

It is not a mere coincidence that none of the studies reviewed by KLERMAN and IZEN have attempted to assess normal vs. atypical grief and thus investigate the hypothesis that the latter increases susceptibility to (psychosomatic) illness.

The authors' conclusion that the evidence is adequate to support the claim of increased mortality among the bereaved seems reasonable and is in agreement with the conclusion of an unpublished review [JACOBS and OSTFELD, in press] which brings in a few more of the most recent studies.

Analyses of mortality rates by marital status [e.g., KRAUS and LILIENFELD, 1959; National Center for Health Statistics, 1970] are not, strictly speaking, bereavement studies since there is no control for length of time since death of spouse. Because the effect of bereavement is most pronounced within the first 2 years (perhaps first 6 months), one would expect such analyses to reflect only diluted effects of bereavement (however, this should be less so among the very young widowed). On the other hand, such analyses also pick up other effects, e.g., the self-selection factors involved in not remarrying or the continued social isolation aspects of not having a spouse (that is, above and beyond the acute effects of the loss experience).

Nevertheless, such analyses provide very useful information – especially if we keep our eyes open on the single and divorced categories as well. For example, the standardized mortality ratios for US 1959–1961 (for all ages and all causes) show the following excess mortality for *widowed* compared to married persons: 45%, white women; 54%, white men; 73%, nonwhite women; 82%, nonwhite men. The excess mortality for *single* persons compared to married ones are, for the same 4 groups, 30, 48, 36 and 52%, respectively. The effects of widowed status are stronger in the younger age categories and weaker in the older age groups, but this *also holds true for the effects of single status* (except for the very youngest age group in such analyses). Mortality due to one cause, arteriosclerotic heart disease, including CHD (ICD No. 420) shows excesses among the widowed which are of about the same magnitude as the overall excess mortality, in all 4 sex-race groups; the same is true for the magnitude of excess mortality among single persons. In short, while it would be too simplistic to argue that the mortality of the widowed should be compared with that of the single, not the married, since this zeroes in more precisely on the experience of bereavement but holds constant the effect of not being married (for example, the self-selection biases must be somewhat different) – nevertheless, the argument does have some merit. And when this is done, the apparent bereavement effects are, of course, much smaller.

Analyses by sex-race and cause of death also reveal interesting differences in the excess mortality among widowed, in comparison to married. For example, the 73% excess in overall mortality among nonwithe women is pretty much like that for all major causes execpt suicide (148% excess); the other 3 sex-race groups show excess mortality due to cancer to ba relatively very small and several other causes (suicide, accidents, TB) to be extra high. In other words, there is an unusually low variability in excess of cause-specific mortality among nonwhite women, suggesting a much more uniform effect of widowed status among them.

(There seems to be a slight error in the author's discussion of table II. The statement (top p. 73) that 'when all these disease groups were combined, the mortality rate was at least 7 times greater...' cannot be right since combining the rates leads back to table I where the values are considerably below 7. Also on that same page, the matching procedure in the REES and LUTKINS study should indicate that the 878 nonbereaved controls were comparable to the 903 bereaved relatives; they were not matched with the decreased.)

The number of published studies dealing with bereavement and mortality is surprisingly small (about 10–12), given the attention this topic has received. Moreover, only about half of these studies have a large enough N to permit adequately reliable estimates. The two studies which found no elevation in mortality [CLAYTON, 1974; WARD, 1976] involved smallish numbers. In general, the effect appears to be greater for men than for women; it may also be grater for younger subjects, but this is firmly established only in the analyses of national vital statistics by marital status. There is some evidence that the greatest period of risk is the first 6 months for men and the first 2 years (the second one more so than the first) for women. Reliable elevations beyond 2 years are not observed (except for suicides among bereaved) and beyond 4–5 years there may be some reduction in mortality below expected.

Both KLERMAN and IZEN, and JACOBS and OSTFELD [in press] offer the reader a number of mechanisms or processes which have been proposed to account for the elevated mortality. The three labelled 'joint unfavorable environment', 'loss of care', and 'desolation effect', are the most plausible ones and it would seem virtually certain that all 3 are operating to some extent. On the basis of the studies reviewed, it is obvious that we have not yet taken even the first step in quantifying their relative contribution. Many variables which influence mortality (socioeconomic status, diet, obesity, alcohol consumption) are shared by spouses and other members of the family, and their effect needs to be estimated.

It is also well to remember that the vital statistics analyses for widowed persons reveal particularly great excess mortality for: motor vehicle accidents, all other accidents, suicide, homicide, and cirrhosis of the liver (all these for men in particular.) These are causes of death where primarily behavioral rather than biological pathways are involved.

The link between bereavement and suicide seems well established. National data [National Center for Health Statistics, 1967] reveal the following excess suicide mortality among the widowed: 66%, white women; 139%, white men; 148%, nonwhite women; and 119%, nonwhite men. White men over 65 who are widowed are at particularly great risk for suicide. It would seem that in this area the evidence is solid enough for us to move beyond mere additional documentation of the relationship and toward a more detailed exploration of the significance of marital, kinship and other social relationships [BOCK, 1972]. One such study is the BOCK and WEBBER (1972) analysis of suicide rates of the elderly in one Florida county. The estimated rates (per 100,000) were as follows: 8.1, married women; 11.0 widowed women, 23.9, married men; 80.7 widowed men. When they also measured the strength of the relational system (organizational membership, location of kin), they found a strong gradient in each sex-marital status category: lower suicide rates for those in a stronger system. Finally, it is worth noting that being widowed was associated with a weaker relational system among the men, but there was no difference for the women.

The evidence which KLERMAN and IZEN review under the heading 'Specific Medical Disorders' (pp. 81–89) is quite uneven and, overall, not yet convincing. Many of the studies do not even particularly deal with bereavement, but with a broader notion of loss or separation and their affective consequences; the methodology of measuring this 'independent' variable is weak. The interpretation that what is being observed is an association between bereavement-loss-separation and onset of some form of medical care (but not of illness) cannot be rejected in many instances. (The evidence for increased health-care seeking behavior following bereavement appears pretty good, as reviewed by KLERMAN and IZEN.)

Self-reports of symptoms and self-assessments of physical health and well-being certainly support the notion of greater felt distress among the bereaved. The manifestations of this distress are varied and are characteristic of the kinds of psychophysiological symptoms typically used in scales measuring depression and anxiety-tension. But it is very difficult to evaluate the significance of these findings: (a) How does one separate in these data, conceptually and methodologically, symptoms indicative of grief itself from symptoms indicative of the consequences of bereavement? (b) The temporal pattern of these symptom elevations is unclear since typically data for only one follow-up occasion are presented. (c) What is the significance of these symptoms for later morbidity and mortality? (d) How does one deal with the whole issue of the 'demand characteristics' of the post-bereavement research interview which encourages the reporting of symptoms?

It is certainly distressing to find that the one study which used the best design – prospective follow-up with initial health evaluation prior to bereavement, which is part of the Duke University aging project – failed to reveal any health deficits attributable to bereavement. The Duke study subjects are somewhat more priviledged socioeconomically, and there may even be social buffer effects due to continued participation in a long-term health study – both of which may contribute to the unrepresentativess of the results. Nevertheless, because of the superior design, these findings must be taken seriously.

Interview-based measurement of health status and well-being is certainly a difficult problem. PARKES [1970], for example, notes in one study that self-assessed health did not correlate with reports of symptoms; however, it did correlate ($r = 0.60$) with interviewers' observations of anger-irritation! The measure of outcome which PARKES [1975] developed in a later report is hardly a methodological advance: coders' ratings of level of functioning, acceptance of reality, withdrawal attitude toward future, physical health, anxiety/depression, and guilt/anger. There are too many problems with such an approach (reliability, validity, implicit weighting, etc.) to make this a useful index, yielding interpretable findings. For example, PARKES reports that lower social-class subjects have poorer outcome; but is there a social class bias in the ratings, or is there an association with social class irrespective of doing any study of bereavement? Moreover, some of the 'predictors' of outcome at 1 year bereavement reaction of severe distress, yearning, anger, self-reproach – are highly similar to what is being measured in the outcome, and thus all one may be observing is the temporal stability of individual differences in these reactions. However, the finding of poorer outcome in connection with short terminal illness and little warning of impending death, appears to be above these methodological critisms.

KLERMAN's and IZEN's discussion of methodological issues is excellent and their call for prospective studies should not go unheeded. In particular, there is a great need to have better initial data on the health status of the bereaved. Health status obtained prior to bereavement is ideal and we need to be more inventive in piggybacking on to existing longitudinal studies (such as cardiovascular surveillance of total communities) or in identifying high risk groups (e.g., spouses of those on critical lists). Other neglected areas are: some documentation of the nature of the relationship with the decreased, and more information on the whole social setting of grieving and recovery.

Migration and Illness
I. PRIOR

The work of PRIOR and his colleagues, exploring the health consequences of migration, is very exciting in the way that it takes advantage of the 'natural experiment' situation. Their design includes very good baseline data on migrants prior to migration and on non-migrants [e.g., PRIOR *et al.*, 1974; STANHOPE and PRIOR, 1976], thus permitting an adequate assessment of initial differences which might point to self-selection factors. Migrants are followed prospectively, thus permitting an assessment of intra-person changes in health status. Careful attention is paid to dietary changes and other behaviors which have probable health consequences, thus taking care of the major criticism in the Ostfeld-D'Atri chapter. And outcome variables include a range of health status indicators collected by an interdisciplinary epidemiological team of physicians and social scientists. In view of the fact that migration is such a complex phenomenon, it is hard to see how a lesser study design can adequately document the health consequences of such an experience. This is not to deny, however, the usefulness of well-executed, cross-sectional studies which have one specific, limited goal, such as the study of differences in acceptance of medical care among recent migrants vs. long term residents [MORGAN, 1973].

Health studies of migrants can be roughly classified into two types: (a) those concerned with the health effects of the experience (which is the focus of PRIOR's chapter) and (b) those concerned with a particular approach to the study of environmental factors in disease. The logic of this latter approach [KAGAN *et al.*, 1974; KMET, 1970] is to start out with known geographical differences in rates of disease (most frequently cancer) and then choose migrant populations which are intended to maximize interpopulation variability in the environmental factors and minimize genetic and other factors (not necessarily known) on which the migrant populations are presumed to be relatively homogeneous.

In some sense, the two types of studies appear to have opposite or incompatible objectives: in the first type, environmental variability is undesirable and complicates the interpretation of differences or changes in health outcomes, while in the second type, any pronounced health effects of the migration experience are bound to be confused with environmental effects. However, what both sets of studies have in common is the absolute need to have some handle on variables which characterize (a) the self-selection of migrants and non-migrants and (b) the intervening processes (adaptation, dietary changes, utilization of health services, etc.). Failure to deal with these variables produces reports which do not add to our knowledge. For example, the MANCUSO and STERLING [1974] analysis of cancer mortality among Ohio residents by place of birth in the US details some excess mortality among those born in the North Eastern and Southern states; but these differences fail to illuminate the original data on geographical differences in US rates by region, and they certainly do not say anything about the health effects of migration. In contrast, the careful work of MARMOT and SYME [1976] reveals: (a) a coronary heart disease gradient among Japanese living in Japan, Hawaii, and the US; (b) differences in dietary intake, serum cholesterol, blood pressure and smoking account for most but not all of this gradient; (c) Japanese-Americans in California who are most traditional have lowest CHD rates, and (d) differences in major coronary risk factors do not account for all of this difference in rates among the Japanese in California.

The articles by MCKINLEY [1975] and WESSEN [1971] serve as a useful introduction to the complex nature of the migration phenomenon. Above all, there seems to be a great deal of specificity about each particular migration: (a) the point in time or stage in the migration process; (b) the sociodemographic composition of the groups involved, and how this may differ with time; (c) the precipitating factors stimulating the migration, and the change in these with time, and (d) the multifaceted nature of the environmental change. The complex influences of these variables would suggest that any health effects observed in a particular study may not be generalizable to other types of migration experiences which may have their own unique characteristics. Moreover, some of the issues which have been raised [WESSEN, 1971] call for measurements of difficult and subtle variables. For example, migrants may differ on sensitivity to environmental change and in adaptability, but these are concepts which are difficult to operationalize.

Theoretical formulations regarding the process have been fairly diverse

[KUO, 1976]. The major ones have emphasized social isolation and cultural 'shock'-cultural change as the major sources of stress with greatest potential for health consequences. Most formulations are rather broad and vague (e.g., CASSEL's 3 hypotheses which form the springboard for Prior's discussion) and greater detail and precision of the theoretical framework underpinning a particular study would make it easier for the reader to evaluate the extent to which the data support a particular theoretical formulation.

However, it seems to me that the greatest obstacle to definitive interpretation of many findings has been the difficulty of linking the actual measures used in a particular study to one or another of the theoretical concepts which are introduced in migration theories. Consider, for example, the frequently used variables such as length of residence in new culture, or first vs. second vs. third generation immigrant status. Length of residence could reflect one or more of the following concepts: (a) length of exposure to the particular environmental effects; (b) the time relationship (delay in effects) between the social change and the particular health outcome; (c) the increase (or decrease?) in social isolation; (d) the decrease (or increase?) in culture 'shock' and culture conflict; (e) the (probable) increase in familiarity with and effectiveness in use of local resources, such as the health care system, and (f) coming early vs. late in the stage of that particular migration process. Given that many conceptual dimensions could be involved, it is difficult to see what is being measured by length of residence, and whether it bears a positive or a negative or a curvilinear association with amount of 'stress'.

SCOTCH [1963], for example, reported that among male Zulus in the urban setting, the longer the residence in the urban setting the higher the blood pressure. (PRIOR incorrectly cites these data [p. 112] as showing lower blood pressure.) But since he generally found that maintenance of traditional cultural practices (which presumably goes down with time) is associated with higher blood pressure, it is difficult to know what to make of it. Italian immigrants living in Australia have lower blood pressure which increases only very slightly with length of residence [ULMAN and ABERNATHY, 1975]; however, their mortality from arteriosclerotic and degenerative heart disease (ICD No. 420–422) goes up strikingly with years of residence [SHEPHERD, 1974]. A better understanding of this complex variable, length of residence, might help us interpret these differential effects.

Even measures specifically developed for a particular migration study are difficult to link to the proper theoretical concept. For example, the 'social interaction' measure developed by PRIOR (amount of interaction with New Zealand institutions and Europeans) is ambiguous regarding its relation to the concept of cultural conflict. High conflict could be experienced by those who have frequent contact with Western ways because each contact represents an instance of a clash between their native and the new values and standards. On the other hand, high conflict could be experienced by those with rare contacts with Western ways, because they are not learning the ways of the new, dominant culture and they experience fear and uncertainty about how to behave and what to expect. Since PRIOR obtained a positive association between amount of social interaction and high blood pressure, he is inclined to view the measure as reflecting high conflict for those with high contact. On the other hand, BEISER *et al.* [1976] report somewhat lower blood pressure among male Serer of Senegal who were high on acculturation (knowledge of and preference for French and Western ways); similarly, SCOTCH [1963] found lower blood pressure among those urban Zulus belonging to Christian churches and attending European clinics.

Are the PRIOR data inconsistent with these 2 studies or are different underlying concepts being measured? It is likely that one and the same measure has a different meaning, depending upon the social setting of the subjects. For example, migrants who live in a social enclave of other migrants from the same region, whose dominant orientation is to retain the old values, and who support each other in the maintenance of old ways – for these subjects, frequent contacts with the dominant culture may mean frequent conflict. On the other hand, migrants who live apart from others like themselves, who aspire toward the ways of the new culture, and who receive no social support from maintenance of old ways – for these subjects frequent contacts may reflect successful and speedy adaptation.

In general, when maintenance of traditional ways is related to lower rates of disease (as in the MARMOT and SYME [1976] study of CHD among Japanese-Americans), there is a tendency to view traditionalism as reflecting social support and buffer against stress; on the other hand, when it is related to higher rates, traditionalism is viewed as indicating high cultural 'shock' and conflict. Thus no matter how the findings come out, we have an 'explanation'. We need a more precise a priori specification of the circumstances under which one or the other interpretation of the measure applies. STRUENING *et al.* [1969] have suggested that 'stress' may be expected to be most intense when (a) the original culture differs radically from the new, (b) there are no available familiar groups to join and modify the intensity of cultural change, and (c) the receiving society most actively emphasizes rapid assimilation. This formulation may help us to move toward such greater specificity.

The overwhelming impression one gains from the migration and health studies is that results do not cohere into a uniform picture. For example, studies using a comparable cross-sectional design [BEISER *et al.*, 1976; BENYOUSEF *et al.*, 1974; LABARTHE *et al.*, 1973; SCOTCH, 1963] did not obtain very comparable differences on blood pressure and other cardiovascular risk factors. It has been difficult to pin down even specific facts, such as: are rural migrants to urban areas less likely to utilize health services [STROMBERG *et al.*, 1974], or are they as receptive (or even more receptive) to modern medical practices as long-standing urban residents [MORGAN, 1973]? But against this background of at best partially replicated findings, there is the strong suggestion that each migration study is somewhat different, examining a different phenomenon in a different setting. Replication of findings, the usual yardstick of trustworthiness of scientific data, then becomes an inapplicable criterion, and we fall back on the other major criterion, quality of research methodology. It is for this reason that PRIOR's work is so important: it uses the most appropriate and probing design for the study of health effects of migration.

It might be noted that sociocultural change, particularly that which is associated with industrialization and urbanization, comes about in two ways: the migrating person makes the change or the environment of the non-migrant changes around him. It is likely that a systematic comparison and contrast of the findings from the two sets of studies (the latter being less common) would prove to be illuminating, particularly regarding the role of such factors as self-selection, social isolation-social support, changes in life style, and the whole process of assimilation-adaptation.

Occupational Mobility and Health
E. BERKANOVIC and P.C. KROCHALK

Many of the comments which I made earlier in the general discussion of the study of social change are particularly relevant when looking at occupational mobility: (a) the importance of the perspective which emphasizes 'normative' change and life cycle orientation; (b) the relevance of the 'person-environment fit' orientation; (c) the need for a dimensionalized environmental description of the change (such as job promotion) rather than an exclusive concern with the experiential aspects of change in general, and (d) the need to utilize the 'natural experiment' approach and to adopt a broad and rich social-psychological perspective on the variables which need to be assessed. Comments which have been made in connection with the study of specific changes (particularly migration) are also highly relevant here. Moreover, since much of the work on occupational mobility deals with CHD, the JENKINS chapter and my discussion of it are also pertinent here.

The relevant evidence on occupational mobility and health is a little more extensive than BERKANOVIC and KROCHALK would lead us to believe. For example, the authors fail to cite some major reports [e.g., LEHMAN *et al.*, 1967] as well as studies which are more difficult to access, such as doctoral dissertations [e.g., WILLIAMS, 1968]. Still other relevant evidence is well hidden in articles which primarily deal with other issues [e.g., JENKINS *et al.*, 1966]. Nevertheless, it is very likely that citation of additional evidence would not have materially altered the major impression, which is that the evidence is limited, not very consistent, and that the problem has been attacked thus far in a most superficial manner. But what is needed is a more incisive view of the problem.

One perspective that is totally missing from the reported studies and the brief review chapter is the approach of the investigator who is concerned with the influence of the work environment on health. (This is comparable to studying migration without any concern for describing the environmental factors in the old and the new settings.) A change in jobs can be analyzed in terms of the change along a set of dimensions that are typically used in investigations of the work environment [e.g., CAPLAN *et al.*, 1975; KAHN *et al.*, 1964; KASL, 1973; QUINN *et al.*, 1971; QUINN and SHEPARD, 1974; ROBINSON *et al.*, 1969]. As suggested earlier, this permits one to analyze rather adequately the differences in the meaning of job promotion, say, for an associate professor to professor vs. a senior engineer in R and D Division moving on to vice-president in sales division. An even more complete way of dimensionalizing and analyzing the nature of the job change is to utilize the 'person-environment fit' perspective [FRENCH, 1974; FRENCH *et al.*, 1974; VAN HARRISON, in press]: the job change can be then seen as the change in the fit between the person characteristics (needs, skills, abilities) and the work environment characteristics (job demands, resources in the job setting, sources of need satisfaction). Coronary-prone behavior pattern type A might be particularly appropriate to study in conjunction with job change; there is some limited evidence [COHEN, 1974] that effects of occupational mobility may interact with type A behavior in affecting CHD rates.

Changes in health status following a job change could be attributed to the fact that the new work setting is associated with greater health risk, rather than to the fact of change *per se*. For example, the job of a foreman appears to be associated with elevated rates of peptic ulcer [PFLANZ, 1971; SUSSER, 1967]; consequently, a higher incidence of peptic ulcers among blue collar workers who became foremen, than among blue collar workers who experienced no job change, would by itself not be a convincing indication of health effects of change *per se*. While the effects of change should diminish over time and the effects of job demands should perhaps cumulate and increase over time, it is still difficult to see how one would disentangle the 2 interpretations. The matter is made even more complicated by the interpretation of the higher rates of ulcers among foremen as being due to the conflicting loyalties and demands experienced by the foreman: they identify with the blue collar workers, from whose ranks they came, but they must also supervise them and identify with management. If it were to be shown that foremen who come in from 'outside' (they were never co-workers with the men they are now supervising) are not at higher risk for ulcers, then it could perhaps be argued that the original observation of higher ulcer rates among foremen is not a general effect of that work environment, but a specific effect among men with a particular occupational mobility pattern.

Another viewpoint that is missing from the studies of occupational mobility and health is the life cycle perspective and the link between mobility and goals and aspirations. It is difficult to see how the meaning and the social context of a particular job change – or lack of job change – can be assessed unless these perspectives are brought in. Theorists such as GROSS [1970], PEPITONE [1967], and PARKER and KLEINER [1966] have offered conceptual frameworks and hypotheses that deal with this issue.

It is clear that the study of occupational mobility and job change is potentially a study of many other changes and influences which can confound causal interpretation. However, this is not unique to this topic (e.g., see the comments on migration) and, depending on the particulars of a research setting, the problems may or may not be serious. What is needed is a close analysis of all the possible changes that have been inadvertently included in the 'experimental treatment', the occupational change. For example, automation and job enlargement may only change the job demands and the work setting; within-company and within-plant transfers, with no change in title, may only alter the social networks and interactions; permanent plant shutdown may precipitate not only job change, but also economic deprivation and breaking up of social networks, depending on the urban vs. rural setting of a plant [GORE, 1973]. Other changes, such as voluntary inter-company moves involving change in company, nature of job, and geographical location are so complex that the influences probably cannot be disentangled; in such situations, the health effects on the whole family should be studied [e.g., OLIVE *et al.*, 1976; WEISSMAN and PAYKEL, 1972].

In general, studies of voluntary job changes and promotions will also have a severe problem with self-selection factors. For example, executives participating in an executive development program (and thus slated for near-future promotion) have higher serum uric acid levels than a group of unselected executives [MONTOYE *et al.*, 1967]; stably higher uric acid levels are also fond among men who, when facing an impending plant shutdown, resign early to find a different job, compared with lower uric acid levels among men who wait for company-scheduled termination [KASL *et al.*, 1968]. Men without college education who nevertheless rise into the executive ranks in the Bell system are quite different (smoking, social background, non-work activities) from their college-educated colleagues [CHRISTENSON and HINKLE, 1961; HINKLE *et al.*, 1966, 1968]. It must be also noted that company promotions practices which favor those in better health would also introduce biases to the study of mobility, which would obscure its effects.

The study of occupational mobility could certainly profit from conceptual clarifications and increased precision of a number of related concepts and ideas, particularly those involving status incongruity and the distinction between inter- and intragenerational mobility. For example, intraperson educational level-occupational status incongruity may take the form of: (a) 'excess' of educational achievement, which could reflect inadequate upward occupational mobility and job demands inadequate to training and abilities, and (b) 'excess' of occupational achievement, which could reflect unusually great upward mobility and job demands exceeding skills and training. In other words, various theoretical and dynamic (developmental) links are possible between concepts of mobility, incongruity, and current person environment fit on job. Moreover, different self-selection factors are probably involved with each developmental pattern. Similarly, interperson status incongruence, such as discrepancy in educational levels of husband and wife (which appears to have implications for CHD [SHEKELLE *et al.*, 1969] and rheumatoid arthritis [KASL and COBB, 1969]) must be linked to other concepts. For example, some forms of spouse pair incongruity have their origins in marital selection, while others may be linked developmentally to one the partner's occupational mobility. Thus, occupational mobility may serve to increase or reduce initial marital status incongruity. Also unexplored is the dynamic relationship among incongruities; for example, is it 'better' (in terms of health outcomes) for a man whose educational level considerably exceeds his occupational attainment to be married to a wife whose educational level is congruent with his educational status or his occupational status?

Theoretical developments concerning intergenerational mobility and its health consequences are even in a more primitive state. For example, we do not know which aspects of the data on social status of family of origin should be treated as indicating a stable predisposition or a vulnerability in the subject, which by itself is of predictive significance, as opposed to which aspects must be examined together with the status data on the subject before their effect becomes apparent (i.e., as a relational construct). In the case-control study of first MIs in a Connecticut county [WARDWELL *et al.,* 1968], it was found that the relative risk associated with 'having trouble relaxing after a hard day' was 4.24. The prevalence of this risk factor by father's occupational level was: upper, 26%; middle, 35%; and lower, 6%. No significant association was found with subject's own occupational status. This pattern of results would seem to suggest that the influence of parental status operates (at least in part) via the creation of a predisposition in the offspring and thus the construction of intergenerational mobility indices may be unnecessary.

Intergenerational mobility indices measure some global aspect of the social distance between family of origin and subject's present situation. Are we to understand that by itself this is a potential predictor of health outcomes, or must we study it in interaction with other factors; and if the latter, what factors? We have noted in conjunction with the migration studies that various measures of exposure to modern ways (knowledge, contact, adoption of practices) probably interact with the social situation of the migrant, i.e., their effects depend upon whether the migrant lives in a social enclave which holds on to the old ways or is already isolated from his original peers and relatives. It is likely that indices of intergenerational mobility show similar situational specificity – or at least a richer theoretical framework would help us think through these issues.

Since social support is quickly coming into its own as an important social factor in health [e.g., COBB, 1976; KAPLAN *et al.,* 1977; PINNEAU, 1976], it is well to note that the effects of occupational mobility may operate via (or may be modified by) social support and changes therein. For example, FRENCH [1974] summarizes some of the NASA study data which tend to show that the association between job stresses (e.g., work load, role ambiguity) and physiological outcomes (blood pressure, serum glucose, and cortisol) is positive among men with poor interpersonal relations with co-workers, supervisors, and subordinates, and absent or negative among men with good interpersonal relations. And in an earlier NASA report [FRENCH and CAPLAN, 1970] they showed that administrators tended to have lower blood pressure in relation to the extent to which their organizational unit involved mostly other administrators and higher blood pressure to the extent that it involved scientists and engineers. CASSEL [1963] had noted that shift workers with a constant set of co-workers had considerably lower cholesterol levels than those whose co-workers were everchanging. And the importance of social interaction on the job as a substitute source of job satisfaction when the work is intrinsically dull and boring has been also noted by those primarily concerned with mental health outcomes [e.g., FORM, 1973; STRAUSS, 1974]. All of these results strongly suggest that the study of job changes should include the study of any changes in social interaction and social support.

In view of the recent documentation that the lower frequency of CHD among men living in Japan, compared to Japanese men living in Hawaii and California, cannot be adequately explained by differences in established risk factors [MARMOT *et al.*, 1975], it is well to look back at MATSUMOTO's [1970] essay which sought to 'explain' the low rates of CHD in Japan. Among the differences between Japanese and American society which he hypothesized might be responsible, the most prominent one was his description of the typical occupational career of a Japanese worker. It would appear that the firm one works for, the work setting, and one's co-workers truly become an extended family, which has enormous stability over time and provides an unchanging order. Work and other activities, such as leisure, become intimately intertwined and possibly a blurring of social roles takes place. This essay is a challenge to investigators of occupational mobility to translate these ideas into researchable hypotheses applicable to the American scene.

Retirement and Health

F.M. CARP

Among the social changes and social situations which are examined in this volume, retirement is undoubtedly the one which is the most institutionalized, i.e., the one which involves the richest network of social and cultural norms and regulations, expectations and practices. In the study of health effects of social change, retirement is perhaps somewhat of a paradox. On the one hand, retirement (as event, or process, or status) can be associated with so many important changes in one's life situation that the potential for adverse health effects should be overwhelming. On the other hand, retirement is so richly embedded in a network of individual and social influences – it can link up with so many variables in the individual's previous life experience, and so many social context and social-institutional determinants – that any hope of being able to trace health changes to retirement *per se* (detect any 'average' effect of retirement) appears small indeed.

CARP, one of the major investigators in the area of retirement, offers us an overview of (a) the rich theoretical formulations which have been developed to study retirement, (b) the methodological and conceptual difficulties in disentangling the mutual influences between health status and retirement, and (c) the evidence which bears on the issue of health consequences of retirement. The last point is organized into 3 sections ('deleterious', 'beneficial', and 'it depends'), undoubtedly in order to present a 'balanced' picture. It is curious that no section entitled 'no demonstrated effects' is included.

The 'evidence' discussed under 'deleterious' effects (pp. 147–150) turns out to contain very little evidence at all. Some of the citations deal with opinions of experts and of clinical observers of the scene, who probably have a very biased exposure to a segment of the phenomenon, i.e., those seeking some help or treatment. The other citations deal with general references to SELYE and LEVI, to studies of various general environmental influences (mostly transient) on cardiovascular functions, and some very global (and optimistic) references to the life events-schedule of recent experience studies. I am not sure how CARP intends the reader to view this section of the review and I am particularly puzzled by her conclusion that 'the sheer scope and pervasiveness of changes *must* forecast physical illness, according to the Holmes and Rahe paradigm' (p. 149); I trust it is a forceful way of stating a hypothesis rather than summarizing any evidence.

It is a paradox that workers in the field of retirement should look to the SRE-type literature in order to augment the viewpoint that retirement may have adverse health consequences. (In this literature – problematic as it is in an overall sense – there is no hope of tractoring any effetcs to a single event, retirement; in fact, the age range of the subjects in the vast majority of the studies would suggest that retirement as an event would very seldom be checked.) One would hope, instead, that workers in the field of life events-SRE would look toward the specific literature on retirement in order to better understand why retirement should be included in or excluded from the list of events.

If one organizes the evidence on retirement the same way as the bereavement literature was examined, then the first question concerns evidence on mortality. The concensus from several studies [FRIEDMAN and ORBACH, 1974; HAYNES, 1975; MCMAHAN and FORD, 1955; MYERS, 1954; TYHURST *et al.*, 1957] is one of no demonstrable elevations in mortality due to retirement. This is in definite contrast to the conclusion coming from the bereavement studies.

HAYNES' [1975] study of united Rubber Workers Union in 2 companies offers perhaps the most thoughtful analysis of the issues, as well as the data. Analyses by year after retirement revealed some peaks during the 3rd and 4th years, with lower rates either during the first 2 years or the 5th through 10th years. But during these 2 peak years, the mortality of the retirees was equal to expected (from actuarial tables) and was lower than expected during the other years; hence, clearly no demonstration of an adverse effect. Moreover, the shapes of the mortality distributions by year postretirement were substantially different in the 2 companies examined, and thus the summary curve does not appear very reliable. Analyses of mortality by year prior to retirement (to test for an anticipation effect just before impending retirement) revealed declining mortality with approaching retirement. This was contrary to the hypothesis, but easily explainable by selective attrition from the work force of those who retired early for health reasons.

The problem of actuarial computation of expected mortality rates for a study cohort has not been fully solved. The 'healthy worker effect' [MCMICHAEL, 1976], i.e., people of any age who are working have a lower age-specific mortality than the total population, is particularly strong beyond age 65 since good health becomes a more powerful factor in continuing work beyond normal retirement. Hence, mortality rates among workers over 65 are a poor basis for computing expected rates. On the other hand, mortality data based on an over-65 population, all of whom are retired, is hardly an adequate control group for estimating retirement effects.

In their review of the retirement literature, FRIEDMAN and ORBACH [1974] favor the interpretation that retirement may be, on the average, beneficial for physical well being. Evidence consistent with this conclusion comes from STREIB and SCHNEIDER [1971], RYSER and SHELDON [1969], BARFIELD and MORGAN [1969], and the studies cited by CARP (p. 150); this effect may be particularly strong among unskilled or lower skilled workers. However, the outcome measures in these studies are 'soft' (self reported health) and some studies have only one-time retrospective assessments of health before and after retirement. The STREIB and SCHNEIDER [1971] report is a good prospective study, but suffered from high (and probably selective) loss to follow-up. Self-report measures of health among the elderly do not correlate too well with physicians' assessment [MADDOX, 1964; STAHL, 1970] and the disparity gets larger with increasing age [VAN ZONNEVELD, 1969]. This lack of association is due to specific biases as well as error; for example, elderly persons with a strong work orientation are likely to be health 'optimists'. Overall, it is best to view these measures as indices of morale and well-being among the elderly. Consequently, this leaves the benefits of retirement on physical health status as yet undemonstrated.

It is likely that the view which is in ascendance is that 'it all depends'. Particularly studies dealing with mental health consequences of retirement [e.g., DONAHUE *et al.,* 1960; RILEY and FONER, 1968; THOMPSON *et al.,* 1960] suggest a variety of outcomes; it is hypothesized that adverse consequences may be seen among those who have a negative advance view of retirement, who are reluctant retirees, and who found intrinsic satisfaction in work. It is estimated that no more than a third of persons who leave the work force experience post-retirement difficulties in the satisfaction and well-being area [BARFIELD and MORGAN, 1969; ATCHLEY, 1975; SHANAS *et al.,* 1968].

This would mean that future studies should concentrate on predictors of post-retirement outcome, rather than trying to establish an overall effect. Prior attitude to retirement looms as the single best predictor [FRIEDMAN and ORBACH, 1974], but it has not been possible to link variations in such attitude to commitment to work and to job satisfaction [e.g., ATCHLEY, 1971; GLAMSER, 1976; GOUDY *et al.,* 1975]. But unless we can link this predictor to other variables, we will end up with a very limited understanding of post-retirement outcomes; i.e., that a negative view of the future later correlates with a negative assessment of the present. This would only indicate a stability of morale and life satisfaction over-time and say nothing about retirement *per se*. It would be analogous to the finding [HAYNES, 1975] that post-retirement mortality within a few years of retirement is higher among workers who have lower education and who had lower pay and less skilled jobs; these are general predictors of higher mortality, whether or not one is studying retirement.

The inability to establish clear cut adverse health effects of retirement may be a surprise to many readers. After all, many writers [e.g., ERIKSON, 1956; FRIEDMAN and HAVINGHURST, 1954; MILLER, 1963; TAUSKY and PIEDMONT, 1967/68] have described work as a central life activity, as a chief source of contact with society at large, as a major influence on self-concept or self-identity – in short, as having many broad 'universal' functions.

If work is so vastly important, should not retirement have correspondingly powerful consequences? But what do the attitudinal studies on importance of work actually tell us, in contrast to the theoretical statements?

In several national surveys of hopes and fears of US adults [CANTRILL and ROLL, 1971], 'good job, congenial work' are mentioned by no more than 6–9% of respondents, and 'unemployment' by 10–14%. In contrast, issues of good (ill) health and better (lower) standard of living, are consistently the two most frequent hopes and fears, with up to 40% of respondents listing them. Findings of highly similar import are reported by CAMPBELL *et al.* [1976]: about 38% of a national sample of respondents rate 'an interesting job' as 'extremely important', in contrast to 70% for 'being in good health', 74% for 'a happy marriage', 67% for 'a good family life', and 62% for 'a good country to live in'. And several studies which have examined the relative contribution of job satisfaction to overall well-being and happiness [CAMPBELL *et al.,* 1976; WESSMAN, 1956; WILSON, 1967] conclude that family life and spare-time activities are clearly more important.

Studies of retirement also offer suggestive data. The results of a Harris poll [HARRIS, 1965] revealed that respondents (especially the younger ones) desire to retire at an earlier age than they actually expect to retire. A later study, using both a national sample and a sample of older (⩾ 60) automobile workers [BARFIELD and MORGAN, 1969], clearly showed that *financial* considerations are of paramount importance in plans for early retirement and that any attachment to the 'work ethic' plays a small role. When given the opportunity to retire early, one third of the workers did so and another third were planning to do so. Among those already retired [HARRIS, 1965], 39% indicated that retirement failed to fulfill their expectations, but less than a quarter of these dissatisfied retirees gave 'miss work' as the reason. In another study of retirees [LOETHER, 1965], the question 'What do you miss most about not working?' was answered by 68% of respondents with either 'nothing at all' or 'my work associates'.

Other studies of 'meaning of work' [DUBIN, 1965; GECHMAN, 1974; KAHN, 1974; MORSE and WEISS, 1955; ORZACK, 1959] suggest that, even though some 73–80% of employed men would apparently continue working in the hypothetical event of an adequate inheritance, only some 9% gave the reason 'because I enjoy work' and another 10% felt that work contributed to their health or self-respect. If they did not work, only 9% would have missed doing something worthwhile. Results with another methodology, in which the respondent is presented with a number of alternative activities and is asked which one he would miss most, suggest that only about 25% of industrial workers are 'job-oriented', that is, they choose the alternative 'a day's work'. This is close to the results of a national time use study [ROBINSON and CONVERSE, 1972] in which some 25% of respondents picked work-related activities as the most satisfying among 'yesterday's' activities.

Overall, it would appear that lower skilled industrial workers have a rather tenous attachment to the work role. They would continue working in the absence of financial needs, not because of any intrinsic satisfaction in work, but because society has not provided any meaningful alternatives. Blue collar workers still 'accept the necessity of work but expect little fulfillment from their specific job' [STRAUSS, 1974a, p. 54]. Much of the theoretical writing on meaning of work in our society, SAYLES and STRAUSS [1966] suggest, is applicable only to workers who do highly skilled and creative work.

CARP's comments regarding 'the urgent need for longitudinal studies...' (p. 155) are, of course, beyond dispute and certainly echo the recommendations of other contributors to this volume. Moreover, as in the case of other topics covered by this volume, the most effective, feasible research designs are not at all self-evident. Random assignment of workers to retirement vs. working beyond 65 (or to early retirement vs. retirement at 65) are probably not feasible. Comparisons of different industries or different work settings which have different retirement policies are certainly possible, but the range of retirement options needs to be adequately broad and the work settings and the people studied must be sufficiently comparable. But one should not ignore such possibilities as random assignment of healthy retired persons to specific part-time work opportunities vs. continued retirement. In all these studies, the role of financial and economic variables must be assessed carefully, for their independent influence on post-retirement health and well-being is likely to be significant and increasing.

Concluding Comments

At this point I do not wish to go through any tightly reasoned, well-documented summary of material presented either in the chapters of the individual contributors or in my own lengthy dicussion chapter. The material is too diverse and the issues too complex to be effectively summarized. Besides, there is a certain inevitability about the conclusions in such a summary, namely: (1) We do not know as much as we thought. (2) A good deal of the evidence is inconclusive and contradictory. (3) Only a few of the studies are beyond reproach methodologically. (4) We need more research, particularly better designed studies.

All of these conclusions do apply, indeed! And they can be even stated with somewhat greater specificity. We need prospective, longitudinal studies of people going through a particular social change experience. We need to collect social-psychological data of great breadth and depth in order to reflect the intricate embeddedness of these events. We need to study intervening behavioral reactions in order to examine adequately the pathway, 'stress' → changes in health-relevant behaviors → illness, and not overemphasize the more frequently studied pathway, 'stress' → changes in biological functions → illness.

But in addition to these points, all of which essentially presuppose that better research methodology leads to a better demonstration of health effects of social events and situations, I also want to emphasize the view that there probably are not as many effects to be demonstrated in the first place. In other words, I believe that in planning future research, we should limit our expectations regarding how powerful the phenomenon is which we are studying; that, in effect, we have been overemphasizing the adverse health consequences of various social events and situations. People's lives are much longer than our studies of them; they get a second, and a third, and a fourth chance to cope and adapt and use the various mechanisms of ego defense; and the adverse effects are likely to be temporary rather than permanent.

Since what we choose to study and how we choose to study it are, in fact, related to our intuitive view of the phenomenon to be examined, this recommended change in attitude should drive us into a more careful, *a priori* analysis of what payoff may be associated with what research setting and research design, and how we can perhaps increase this payoff with suitable design changes. And that is the intent of this recommended change in attitude.

Part of this more probing analysis should involve a closer scrutiny of the conceptual extrapolation from limited situations of acute stress to broad-range (real-life) situations of chronic stress. The following schema may be helpful in such an analysis.

In cell *A* we have the kind of a situation in which the stress is relatively brief and the stress response extinguishes with repetition of stimulus; such extinction (habituation), moreover, does not seem to require any kind of an active participation on the part of the organism. The prototype situation here is, for example, the evidence that mere approach of a doctor in a

Reactions			
Nature of situational stress	Habituation (passive learning)	Adaptation – coping (psychological-behavioral, physiological)	No adaptation possible or apparent
Intermittent and/or self-limiting	A	C	E
Chronic	B	D	F

hospital may initiate a rise in the blood pressure of a patient [RICHARDSON *et al.*, 1964]; repeated presentation of the same stimulus reduces this response but does not require any active coping on the patient's part. Moreover, such stimuli are only intermittent and for the duration of the hospitalization. The literature on situational influences on blood pressure is replete with evidence of this kind [BENSON and GUTMAN, 1974; OSTFELD and SHEKELLE, 1967], but it is very doubtful that such studies provide much of a basis for extrapolating to situations where we expect to observe long-term changes.

In cell *B* we have a somewhat different situation in that the presentation of the stress stimulus is over an indefinite time span. Studies of effects of residential noise on sleep [e.g., KRYTER, 1972; TARNAPOLSKY and MCLEAN, 1976] are an example: residents living in areas of high noise (subway, airport) generally habituate to this stimulus and such noise loses awakening power. They will still awaken to the noise if it departs from its usual quality (e.g., atypical noise of jet engines upon approach to airport), but that is partly because of the new psychological meaning of the noise. However, noise also interferes with certain daily activities, such as conversation, and there is no habituation effect here.

In cell *C* we are dealing conceptually with the kind of situation where certain behaviors or certain attitudes on the part of the organism, when present, will modify or eliminate the stress reaction. For example, laboratory studies of acute exposure to noise [REIM *et al.*, 1971] and electric shock [GEER *et al.*, 1970] suggest that the mere perception of ability to control aversive stimuli – even if it is never implemented and is, in fact, nonveridical – reduces or eliminates the stress effect, such as increased skin conductance or decreased task performance.

Of course, it may be difficult to know whether the situation under scrutiny belongs in cell *C* or cell *E*. For example, airline pilots show increased heart rate during and after take-off [SMITH, 1967] and this seems to happen irrespective of their length of flying experience; there is no apparent heart rate elevation in flight, but there may be some at approach and landing, depending upon weather conditions. Military pilots of high performance single engine jets [ROMAN, 1963] show elevated blood pressure throughout flight, and particularly so at take-off and landing. In another study [RUBIN, 1974] the levels of serum cortisol were assessed on pilots and radar intercept officers on jet fighter bombers landing on aircraft carriers. (One can hardly think of a more demanding and dangerous task than this.) Results elevated levels only among the pilots; the radar officers, though equally exposed to the danger, are not involved in piloting the plane and did not show higher levels. In a study of 17-OHCS levels in a combat situation [BOURNE *et al.*, 1968], on the day of anticipated attack the officer and the radio operator showed an increase in corticosteroid levels, while the enlisted men showed a decrease. Yet, presumably the soldiers are at least in as great a danger during battle as are the officer and the radio operator. All of these studies would seem to suggest that it is possible to adapt to situations of even extreme physical danger. But if such situations also involve responsibility for certain activities and people, and the need to remain vigilant while performing various tasks, then adaptation may not be possible, no matter how repeated the exposure.

The type of a situation which belongs in cell *D* could be illustrated from many studies. For example, KAHN *et al.* [1964] found that men in management jobs which involved a good deal of chronic role conflict and role overload did not necessarily experience job tension, provided they tended to be rigid and coped by reducing communication with others. School children living in chronically crowded physical conditions with lack of privacy did not show decrement in school achievement, provided the families coped by setting aside time when a particular room was devoted only to quiet pursuits [MICHELSON, 1970].

The type of situation represented by cell *F* is essentially the one with greatest probable payoff for investigators in the field of social stress and disease. From the results of the report on air traffic controllers [COBB and ROSE, 1973] it would appear that this may be a work situation of chronic stress with little possibility of adaptation because of responsibility for people and the need to maintain constant vigilance. Other jobs, such as those involving machine-paced work and skilled judgments which must be made at very short intervals, may also lead to stress reactions without adaptation [FRANKENHAUSER and GARDELL, 1976] but data on long-term effects are not yet available.

The point of offering the above schema is only to stimulate and facilitate analysis of the social stress situation under investigation at the earliest possible point in planning research. The schema is intended for no other purpose. None of the boundaries in this schema can be defined precisely. For example, the distinction between cells *D* and *F* may be sometimes defined in situational terms, but at other times in terms of characteristics of individuals which facilitate or prevent coping; i.e., in a single study, the investigator may have subgroups of individuals in cell *D* and others in cell *F*. Similarly, the distinction between cells *E* and *F* may sometimes be difficult to make. A chronically stressful job situation may be viewed as intermittent stress provided the person can isolate himself from the influences of the work environment when he is not working; but it may be viewed as chronic stress if the person rates, say, high on behavior type A or if his home environment is one of low social support.

Stress reactions identified in situations which belong in cell *A* may, on occasion, be predictive of long-term disease outcomes. The likely reason for this would be that the acute, self-limited stress reaction is an indicator of a generalized reactivity (or of a stable person characteristic) which is predictive of that reaction in a great variety of situations and circumstances. This is, of course, a perfectly interesting and useful predictor of disease, but should not be misinterpreted as revealing the influence of a specific situational stress.

In searching for research opportunities with the greatest probable payoffs, we are not only trying to locate significant social events and situations (those which could be reasonably placed in cells *D*, *E* and *F* in the above schema), but also the optimal time spans in which to make our observations. And here again, we need to be more thoughtful about the issues involved. For most of the social events and situations discussed in the present volume, the optimal time span appears to be one which encompasses the period prior to the event (to collect pre-stress data and to assess anticipation effects) and which follows the person through the various stages of the experience and of adapting to it. This is a difficult and expensive design in which the optimal lenght of following the subjects through a particular experience may not always be clear. But the easier alternatives are really more expensive if they reveal little or nothing. We have too many studies which tell us too little because they are cross-sectional slices of the phenomenon at a very late stage: most of the effects have already taken place and because of these effects, the initial cohort has scattered in so many different ways that the subjects we do catch later in our cross-sectional net are no longer able to help us to reconstruct the experience and its effects.

References

ABERT, J.G. and KAMRASS, M.: Social experiments and social program evaluation (Balinger, Cambridge 1974).

APPLEY, M.H. and TRUMBULL, R.: On the concept of psychological stress; in APPLEY and TRUMBULL Psychological stress, pp. 1–13 (Appleton-Century-Crofts, New York 1967).

ATCHLEY, R.C.: Retirement and work orientation. Gerontologist *11:* 29–32 (1971).

ATCHLEY, R.C.: Adjustment to loss of job at retirement. Int. J. Aging hum. Dev. *6:* 17–27 (1975).

BARFIELD, R. and MORGAN, J.N.: Early retirement: the decision and the experience (Institute for Social Research, The University of Michigan, Ann Arbor 1969).

BARIC, L.: Recognition of the 'at-risk' role. A means to influence health behavior. Int. J. Hlth Educ. *12:* 24–34 (1969).

BECKER, M.H.: The health belief model and personal health behavior. Hlth Educ. Monogr. *2:* 326–473 (1974).

BEISER, M.; COLLOMB, H.; RAVEL, J.L., and NAFZIGER, C.J.: Systemic blood pressure studies among the Serer of Senegal. J. chron. Dis. *29:* 371–380 (1976).

BENNETT, C.A. and LUMSDAINE, A.A.: Evaluation and experiment (Academic Press, New York 1975).

BENSON, H. and GUTMANN, M.C.: The relation of environmental factors to systemic arterial hypertension; in ELIOT Stress and the heart, pp. 13–31 (Futura, Mt. Kisco 1974).

BENYOUSSEF, A.; CUTLER, J.L.; LEVINE, A.; MANSOURIAN, P.; PHAN-TAN, T.; BAYLET, R.; COLLOMB, H.; DIOP, S.; LACOMBE, B.; RAVEL, J.; VAUGELADE, J., and DIEBOLD, G.: Health effects of rural-urban migration in developing countries – Senegal. Soc. Sci. Med. *8:* 243–254 (1974).

BIRLEY, J.L.T. and CONNOLLY, J.: Life events and physical illness; in HILL Modern trends in psychosomatic medicine, vol. 3, pp. 154–165 (Butterworths, London 1976).

BOCK, E.W.: Aging and suicide. The significance of marital, kinship, and alternative relations. Family Coordinat. *1972:* 71–79.

BOCK, E.W. and WBBER, I.L,: Suicide among the elderly: isolating widowhood and mitigating alternatives. Marriage Family *34:* 24–31 (1972).

BONNER, K.: Industrial implications of stress; in LEVI Emotional stress, pp. 225–232 (American Elsevier, New York 1967).

BOURNE, P.G.; ROSE, R.M., and MASON, J.W.: 17-OHCS levels in combat. Archs gen. Psychiat. *19:* 135–140 (1968).

BRAND, R.J.; ROSENMAN, R.H.; SHOLTZ, R.I., and FRIEDMAN, M.: Multivariate prediction of coronary heart disease in the Western Collaborative Group Study compared to the findings of the Framingham study. Circulation *53:* 348–355 (1976).

BROWN, G.W.: Meaning, measurement, and stress of life events; in DOHRENWEND and DOHRENWEND Stressful life events: their nature and effects, pp. 217–243 (Wiley, New York 1974).

BRUCH, H.: Eating disturbances in adolescence; in ARIETI American handbook of Psychiatry, vol. 2, pp. 275–286 (Basic Books, New York 1974).

BRUCH, H.: Anorexia nervosa; in ARIETI American handbook of psychiatry, vol. 4, pp. 787–809 (Basic Books, New York 1975).

BRUHN, J.G.; WOLF, S.; LYNN, T.N.; BIRD, H.B., and CHANDLER, B.: Social aspects of coronary heart disease in a Pennsylvania German community. Soc. Sci. Med. *2:* 201–212 (1968).

BUELL, P. and BRESLOW, L.: Mortality from coronary heart disease in California men who work long hours. J. chron. Dis. *11:* 615–626 (1960).

CAMPBELL, A.; CONVERSE, P.E., and RODGERS, W.L.: The quality of American life (Russell Sage Foundation, New York 1976).

CAMPBELL, D.T.: Reforms as experiments. Am. Psychol. *24:* 409–429 (1969).

CANTRIL, A.H. and ROLL, C.W., jr.: Hopes and fears of the American people (Universe Books, New York 1971).

CAPLAN, R.D.: Organizational stress and individual strain. A social-psychological study of risk factors in coronary heart disease among administrators, engineers, and scientists; unpubl. doct. diss. The University of Michigan, Ann Arbor (1971).

CAPLAN, R.D.: A less heretical view of life change and hospitalization. J. psychosom. Res. *19:* 247–250 (1975).

CAPLAN, R.D.; COBB, S.; FRENCH, J.R.P., jr.; HARRISON, R.V., and PINNEAU, S.R., jr.: Job demands and worker health. HEW Publication No. (NIOSH), pp. 75–160 (Washington 1975).

CAPORASO, J.A. and ROOS, L.L., jr.: Quasi-experimental approaches (Northwestern University Press, Evanston 1973).

CASSEL, J.C.: The use of medical records. Opportunity for epidemiological studies. J. occup. Med. *5:* 185–190 (1963).

CASSEL, J.C.: Psychiatric epidemiology; in ARIETI American handbook of psychiatry, vol. 2, pp. 401–410 (Basic Books, New York 1974).

CASSEL, J.: An epidemiological perspective of psychosocial factors in disease etiology. Am. J. publ. Hlth *64:* 1040–1043 (1974a).

CASSEL, J.: Hypertension and cardiovascular disease in migrants. A potential source of clues? Int. J. Epidem. *3:* 204–206 (1974b).

CASSEL, J.: Social science in epidemiology. Psychosocial processes and 'stress' theoretical formulation; in STRUENING and GUTTENTAG Handbook of evaluation research, vol. 1, pp. 537–549 (Sage Publications, Beverly Hills 1976).

CHEN, E. and COBB, S.: Family structure in relation to health and disease. J. chron. Dis. *12:* 545–567 (1960).

CHRISTENSON, W.N. and HINKLE, L.E., jr.: Differences in illness and prognostic signs in two groups of young men. J. Am. med. Ass. *177:* 247–253 (1961).

CLAYTON, P.J.: Mortality and morbidity in the first year of widowhood. Archs gen. Psychiat. *30:* 747–750 (1974).

COBB, S.: The frequency of rheumatic diseases (Harvard University Press, Cambridge 1971).

COBB, S.: Social support as a moderator of life stress. Psychosom. Med. *38:* 300–314 (1976).

COBB, S. and ROSE, R.M.: Hypertension, peptic ulcer, and diabetes in air traffic controllers. J. Am. med. Ass. *224:* 489–492 (1973).

COHEN, J.B.: Sociocultural change and behavior patterns in disease etiology. An epidemiologic study of coronary disease among Japanese Americans; unpubl. Ph.D. diss. University of California, Berkeley (1974).

COOK, T.D. and CAMPBELL, D.T.: The design and conduct of quasi-experiments and true experiments in field settings; in DUNNETTE Handbook of industrial and organizational psychology, pp. 223–326 (Rand McNally, Chicago 1976).

COOPER, C.L. and MARSHALL, J.: Occupational sources of stress: a review of the literature relating to coronary heart disease and mental ill health. J. occup. Psychol. *49:* 11–28 (1976).

CRISP, A.N.: Psychological aspects of some disorders of weight; in HILL Modern trends in psychosomatic medicine, vol. 2, pp. 124–146 (Appleton-Century-Crofts, New York 1970).

CROOG, S.H. and LEVINE, S.: Social status and subjective perceptions of 250 men after myocardial infarction. Publ. Hlth Rep., Wash. *84:* 989–997 (1969).

DOHRENWEND, B.S.: Multicomponent measurement of the magnitude of stressful life events. An unpublished manuscript (1977).

DOHRENWEND, B.S. and DOHRENWEND, B.P.: Stressful life events: their nature and effects (Wiley, New York 1974).

DONAHUE, W.; ORBACH, H.L., and POLLACK, O.: Retirement: the emerging social pattern; in TIBBITTS Handbook of social gerontology, pp. 330–406 (The University of Chicago Press, Chicago 1960).

DUBIN, R.: Industrial workers' worlds. A study of the 'central life interests' of industrial workers. Soc. Probl. *3:* 131–142 (1956).

DWYER, J.T.; FELDMAN, J.J., and MAYER, J.: The social psychology of dieting. J. Hlth soc. Behav. *11:* 269–287 (1970).

EASTWOOD, M.R.: Epidemiologic studies in psychosomatic medicine. Int. J. psychiat. Med. *6:* 123–132 (1975).

ENGEL, G.L.: Psychological development in health and disease (Saunders, Philadelphia 1962).

ERIKSON, E.H.: The problem of ego identity. J. Am. psychoanal. Ass. *4:* 56–121 (1956).

FEINSTEIN, A.R.: Clinical epidemiology. Ann. intern. Med. *69:* 807–820, 1037–1061, 1287–1312 (1968).

FORM, W.H.: Auto workers and their machines. A study of work, factory and job dissatisfaction in four countries. Soc. Forces *52:* 1–15 (1973).

FRANKENHAEUSER, M. and GARDELL, B.: Underload and overload in working life. Outline of a multidisciplinary approach. J. hum. Stress *2:* 35–46 (1976).

FRENCH, J.R.P., jr.: Person role fit; in MCLEAN Occupational stress, pp. 70–79 (Thomas, Springfield 1974).

FRENCH, J.R.P., jr. and CAPLAN, R.D.: Psychosocial factors in coronary heart disease. Industr. Med. Surg. *39:* 383–397 (1970).

FRENCH, J.R.P., jr.; RODGERS, W., and COBB, S.: Adjustment as person-environment fit; in COELHO, HAMBURG and ADAMS Coping and adaptation, pp. 316–333 (Basic Books, New York 1974).

FRIEDMAN, E.W. and HAVINGHURST, R.J.: The meaning of work and retirement (The University of Chicago Press, Chicago 1954).

FRIEDMAN, E.H. and HELBERSTEIN, H.K.: Occupational stress, law school hierarchy and coronary artery disease in Cleveland attorneys. Psychosom. Med. *30:* 72–86 (1968).

FRIEDMAN, M. and ROSENMAN, R.H.: Type A behavior and your heart (Knopf, New York 1974).

FRIEDMAN, M.; ROSENMAN, R.H., and CARROLL, V.: Changes in serum cholesterol and blood clotting time in men subjected to cyclic variation of occupational stress. Circulation *17:* 852–861 (1958).

FRIEDMAN, E.A. and ORBACH, H.L.: Adjustment to retirement; in ARIETI American handbook of psychiatry, vol. 1, pp. 609–645 (Basic Books, New York 1974).

GECHMAN, A.S.: Without work, life goes... J. occup. Med. *16:* 749–751 (1974).

GEER, J.H.; DAVISON, G.C., and GATCHEL, R.I.: Reduction of stress in humans through nonveridical perceived control of aversive stimulation. J. pers. soc. Psychol. *16:* 731–738 (1970).

GLAMSER, F.D.: Determinants of a positive attitude toward retirement. J. Geront. *31:* 104–107 (1976).

GLASS, D.C.; SNYDER, M.L., and HOLLIS, J.F.: Time urgency and type A coronary-prone behavior pattern. J. appl. soc. Psychol. *4:* 125–140 (1974).

GORE, S.: The influence of social support in ameliorating the consequences of job loss; unpubl. Ph.D. diss. The University of Michigan, Ann Arbor (1973).

GOUDY, W.J.; POWERS, E.A., and KEITH, P.: Work and retirement. A test of attitudinal relationships. J. Geront. *30:* 193–198 (1975).

GRAHAM, S.: The sociological approach to epidemiology. Am. J. publ. Hlth *64:* 1046–1049 (1974).

GROEN, J.J.: Social change and psychosomatic disease; in LEVI Society, stress, and disease, vol. 1, pp. 91–109 (Oxford University Press, London 1971).

GOEN, J.J.: Psychosomatic aspects of ischemic (coronary) heart disease; in HILL Modern trends in psychosomatic medicine, vol. 3, pp. 288–329 (Butterworths, London 1976).

GROEN, J.J. and BASTIAANS, J.: Psychosocial stress, interhuman communication, and psychosomatic disease; in SPIELBERGER and SARASON Stress and anxiety, vol. 1, pp. 27–49 (Hemisphere Publishing Corp., Washington 1975).

GROEN, J.J. and DRORY, S.: Influence of psychosocial factors on coronary heart disease. Path. Microbiol. *30:* 779–788 (1967).

GROSS, E.: Work, organization, and stress; in LEVINE and SCOTCH Social stress, pp. 54–110 (Aldine, Chicago 1970).

GURALNICK, L.: Mortality by occupation and cause of death (No. 3), Mortality by industry and cause of death (No. 4), Mortality by occupational level and cause of death (No. 5) among men 20 to 64 years of age, U.S. 1950. USDHEW, PHS, Vital Statistics-Special Reports, vol. 53 (1963).

HATANO, S.; SHIGEMATSU, I., and STRASSER, T.: Hypertension and stroke control in the community (WHO, Geneva 1976).

HAYNES, S.G.: Mortality around retirement and the socio-medical correlates of early death among retirees in the rubber industry; unpubl. doct. diss. University of North Carolina, Chapel Hill (1975).

Hill, O.W.: Modern trends in psychosomatic medicine, vol. 2 (Appleton-Century-Crofts, New York 1970).

Hill, O.: Modern trends in psychosomatic medicine, vol. 3 (Butterworths, London 1976).

Hill, O.H.: Anorexia nervosa; in Hill Modern trends in psychosomatic medicine, vol. 3, pp. 382–403 (Butterworths, London 1976).

Hinkle, L.E., jr.: The effect of exposure to culture change, social change, and changes in interpersonal relationships on health; in Dohrenwend and Dohrenwend Stressful life events: their nature and effects, pp. 9–44 (Wiley, New York 1974).

Hinkle, L.E., jr.; Benjamin, B.; Christenson, W.N., and Ullmann, D.S.: Coronary heart disease. Archs envir. Hlth *13:* 312–321 (1966).

Hinkle, L.E., jr.; Dohrenwend, B.P.; Elinson, J.; Kasl, S.V.; McDowell, A.; Mechanic, D., and Syme, L.S.: Social determinants of human health; in preventive medicine, pp. 89–146 (Prodist, New York 1976).

Hinkle, L.E., jr.; Whitney, L.H.; Lehman, E.W.; Dunn, J.; Benjamin, B.; King, R.; Plakun, A., and Fehinger, B.: Occupation, education, and coronary heart disease. Science *161:* 238–246 (1968).

Holmes, T.H. and Masuda, M.: Life change and illness susceptibility; in Dohrenwend and Dohrenwend Stressful life events: their nature and effects, pp. 45–72 (Wiley, New York 1974).

Horan, P.M. and Gray, B.H.: Status inconsistency, mobility, and coronary heart disease. J. Hlth soc. Behav. *15:* 300–310 (1974).

House, J.S.: The relationship of intrinsic and extrinsic work motivations to occupational stress and coronary heart disease risk; unpubl. doct. diss. The University of Michigan, Ann Arbor (1972).

House, J.S.: Occupational stress and coronary heart disease. A review and theoretical integration. J. Hlth soc. Behav. *15:* 12–27 (1974).

Jacobs, S. and Ostfeld, A.M.: An epidemiological review of the mortality of bereavement. Psychosom. Med. (in press).

Jenkins, C.D.: Psychologic and social precursors of coronary disease. New Engl. J. Med. *284:* 244–255, 307–317 (1971).

Jenkins, C.D.: Social and epidemiologic factors in psychosomatic medicine. Psychiat. Ann. *2:* 8–21 (1972).

Jenkins, C.D.: Recent evidence supporting psychologic and social risk factors for coronary disease. New. Engl. J. Med. *294:* 987–994, 1033–1038 (1976).

Jenkins, C.D.; Rosenman, R.H., and Friedman, M.: Components of the coronary-prone behavior pattern. Their relation to silent myocardial infarction and blood lipids. J. chron. Dis. *19:* 599–609 (1966).

Jenkins, C.D.; Rosenman, R.H., and Zyzanski, S.J.: Prediction of clinical coronary heart disease by a test for the coronary-prone behavior pattern. New. Engl. J. Med. *290:* 1271–1275 (1974).

Jenkins, C.D.; Zyzanski, S.J., and Rosenman, R.H.: Progress toward validation of a computer-scored test for type A coronary-prone behavior pattern. Psychosom. Med. *33:* 193–202 (1971).

Jenkins, C.D.; Zyzanski, S.J., and Rosenman, R.H.: Risk of new myocardial infarction in middle-aged men with manifest coronary heart disease. Circulation *53:* 342–347 (1976).

KAGAN, A.: Epidemiology and society, stress and disease; in LEVI Society, stress, and disease, vol. 1, pp. 36–48 (Oxford University Press, London 1971).

KAGAN, A.; HARRIS, B.R.; WINKELSTEIN, W., jr.; JOHNSON, K.G.; KATO, H.; SYME, S.L.; RHOADS, G.G.; GAY, M.L.; NICHAMAN, M.Z.; HAMILTON, H.B., and TILLOTSON J.: Epidemiologic studies of coronary heart disease and stroke in Japanese men living in Japan, Hawaii, and California. Demographic, physical, dietary and biochemical characteristics. J. chron. Dis. *27:* 345–364 (1974).

KAHN, R.L.: On the meaning of work. J. occup. Med. *16:* 716–719 (1974).

KAHN, R.L.; WOLFE, D.M.; QUINN, R.P.; SNOEK, J.D., and ROSENTHAL, R.A.: Organizational stress: studies in role conflict and ambiguity (Wiley, New York 1964).

KAPLAN, B.H.; CASSEL, J.C., and GORE, S.: Social support and health. Med, Care *15:* suppl. 5, pp. 47–58 (1977).

KAPLAN, B.H.; CASSEL, J.C.; TYROLER, H.A.; CORNONI, J.C.; KLEINBAUM, D.G., and HAMES, C.G.: Occupational mobility and coronary heart disease. Archs intern. Med. *128:* 938–942 (1971).

KASL, S.V.: Physical and mental health effects of involuntary relocation and institutionalization on the elderly. – A review. Am. J. Publ. Hlth *62:* 377–384 (1972).

KASL, S.V.: Mental health and the work environment. An examination of the evidence. J. occup. Med. *15:* 509–518 (1973).

KASL, S.V.: Social-psychological characteristics associated with behaviors which reduce cardiovascular risk; in ENELOW and HENDERSON Applying behavioral science to cardiovascular risk, pp. 173–190 (American Heart Association, New York 1975).

KASL, S.V.: Effects of housing on mental and physical health; in Housing in the Seventies Working Papers. 1. National Housing Policy Review, pp. 286–304 (US Department of Housing and Urban Development, Washington 1976).

KASL, S.V.: Effect of involuntary relocation and housing on health. Presented at the Epidemiology of Aging Conference, NIH, Bethesda 1977.

KASL, S.V.: Stress at work. Epidemiological contributions to the study of work stress; in COOPER and PAYNE Stress at work (Wiley, New York, in press).

KASL, S.V. and COBB, S.: Health behavior, illness behavior and sick role behavior. Archs Envir. Hlth *12:* 246–266, 531–541 (1966).

KASL, S.V. and COBB, S.: The intrafamilial transmission of rheumatoid arthritis. VI. Association of rheumatoid arthritis with several types of status inconsistency. J. chron. Dis. *22:* 259–278 (1969).

KASL, S.V.; COBB, S., and BROOKS, G.W.: Changes in serum uric acid and serum cholesterol in men undergoing job loss. J. Am. med. Ass. *206:* 1500–1507 (1968).

KENNY, D.A.: A quasi-experimental approach to assessing treatment effects in nonequivalent control group design. Psychol. Bull. *82:* 345–362 (1975).

KEYS, A.; BROZEK, J.; HENSCHEL, A.; MICKELSON, O., and TAYLOR, H.L.: The biology of human starvation (University of Minnesota Press, Minneapolis 1950).

KMET, J.: The role of migrant population in studies of selected cancer sites. A review. J. chron. Dis. *23:* 305–324 (1970).

KRAUS, A.S. and LILIENFELD, A.M.: Some epidemiologic aspects of the high mortality rate in the young widowed group. J. chron. Dis. *10:* 207–217 (1959).

KRYTER, K.D.: Non-auditory effects of environmental noise. Am. J. publ. Hlth *62:* 389–398 (1972).

KULLER, L.H.: Epidemiology of cardiovascular diseases. Current perspectives. Am. J. Epidem. *104:* 425–456 (1976).

KUO, W. Theories of migration and mental health. An empirical testing on Chinese-Americans. Soc. Sci. Med. *10:* 297–306 (1976).

LABARTHE, D.; REED, D.; BRODY, J., and STALLONES, R.: Health effects of modernization in Palau. Am. J. Epidem. *98:* 161–174 (1973).

LAHORGUE, Z.: Morbidity and marital status. J. chron. Dis. *12:* 476–498 (1960).

LANDY, F.J. and TRUMBO, D.A.: Psychology of work behavior (Dorsey Press, Homewood 1976).

LAZARUS, R.S.: Psychological stress and the coping process (McGraw-Hill, New York 1966).

LAZARUS, R.S.: The concepts of stress and disease; in LEVI Society, stress and disease, vol. 1, pp. 53–58 (Oxford University Press, London 1971).

LEHMAN, E.W.; SCHULMAN, J., and HINKLE, L.E., jr.: Coronary deaths and organizational mobility. Archs Envir. Hlth *15:* 455–461 (1967).

LIPOWSKI, Z.J.: Psychosomatic medicine in a changing society. Some current trends in theory and research. Compreh. Psychiat. *14:* 203–215 (1973).

LIPOWSKI, Z.J.: Physical illness, the patient, and his environment. Psychosocial foundations in medicine; in REISER Organic disorders and psychosomatic medicine. American handbook of psychiatry, vol. 4, pp. 3–42 (Basic Books, New York 1975).

LIPOWSKI, Z.J.: Psychosomatic medicine: an overview; in HILL Modern trends in Psychosomatic medicine, vol. 3, pp. 1–20 (Butterworths, London 1976).

LITMAN, T.J.: The family as a basic unit in health and medical care. A social-behavioral overview. Soc. Sci. Med. *8:* 495–519 (1974).

LOETHER, H.J.: The meaning of work and adjustment to retirement; in SHOSTAK and GOMBERG Blue collar world, pp. 525–533 (Prentice-Hall, Englewood Cliffs 1965).

MACMAHON, B. and PUGH, T.F.: Epidemiology: principles and methods (Little Brown, Boston 1970).

MCGRATH, J.E.: A conceptual formulation for research on stress; in MCGRATH Social and psychological factors in stress, pp. 10–21 (Holt, Rinehart & Winston, New York 1970).

MCGRATH, J.E.: Stress and behavior in organizations; in DUNNETTE Handbook of industrial and organizational psychology, pp. 1351–1395 (Rand McNally, Chicago 1976).

MCKINLEY, J.B.: Some issues associated with migration, health status, and the use of health services. J. chron. Dis. *28:* 579–592 (1975).

MCMAHAN, C.A. and FORD, T.A.: Surviving the first five years after retirement. J. Geront. *10:* 212–215 (1955).

MCMICHAEL, A.J.: Standardized mortality ratios and the 'healthy worker effect'. Scratching beneath the surface. J. occup. Med. *18:* 165–168 (1976).

MADDOX, G.L.: Self-assessment of health status. A longitudinal study of selected elderly subjects. J. chron. Dis. *17:* 449–460 (1964).

MANCUSO, T.P. and STERLING, T.D.: Relation of place of birth and migration in cancer mortality in the U.S. A study of Ohio residents (1959–1967). J. chron. Dis. *27:* 459–474 (1974).

MARMOT, M.G. and SYME, S.L.: Acculturation and coronary heart disease in Japanese-Americans. Am. J. Epidem. *104:* 225–247 (1976).

MARMOT, M.G.; SYME, S.L.; KAGAN, A.; KATO, H.; COHEN, J.B., and BELSKY, J.: Epidemiologic studies of coronary heart disease and stroke in Japanese men living in Japan, Hawaii, and California. Prevalence of coronary and hypertensive heart disease and associated risk factors. Am. J. Epidem. *102:* 514–525 (1975).

MATSUMOTO, Y.S.: Social stress and coronary heart disease in Japan. A hypothesis. Milbank meml Fund q. Bull. *48:* 9–36 (1970).

MAUSNER, J.S. and BAHN, A.K.: Epidemiology: an introductory text (Saunders, Philadelphia 1974).

MECHANIC, D.: Medical sociology (The Free Press, New York 1968).

MECHANIC, D.: Social psychological factors affecting the presentation of bodily complaints. New Engl. J. Med. *286:* 1132–1139 (1972).

MECHANIC, D.: Discussion of research programs on relations between stressful life events and episodes of physical illness; in DOHRENWEND and DOHRENWEND Stressful life events: their nature and effects, pp. 87–97 (Wiley, New York 1974).

MEDALIE, J.H.; SNYDER, M.; GROEN, J.J.; NEUFELD, H.N.; GOLDBOURT, U., and RISS, E.: Angina pectoris among 10,000 men. Am. J. Med. *55:* 583–594 (1973).

METTLIN, C.: Occupational careers and the prevention of coronary-prone behavior. Soc. Sci. Med. *10:* 367–372 (1976).

MICHELSON, W.: Man and his urban environment: A sociological approach (Addison-Wesley, Reading 1970).

MILLER, D.R.: The study of social relationships. Situation, identy, and social interaction; in KOCH Psychology: a study of a science, vol. 5, pp. 639–737 (McGraw-Hill, New York 1963).

MONTOYE, H.J.; FAULKNER, J.A.; DODGE, H.J.; MIKKELSEN, W.M.; WILLIS, P.W., III., and BLOCK, W.D.: Serum uric acid concentrations among business executives. Ann. intern. Med. *66:* 838–850 (1967).

MORGAN, R.W.: Migration as a factor in the acceptance of medical care. Soc. Sci. Med. *7:* 865–873 (1973).

MORSE, N.E. and WEISS, R.S.: The function and meaning of work and the job. Am. sociol. Rev. *20:* 191–198 (1955).

MUELLER, E.F.: Psychological and physiological correlates of work overload among university professors; unpubl. doct. diss. The University of Michigan, Ann Arbor (1965).

MUSTACCHI, P.: Arterial hypertension and the work environment. Some considerations affecting its compensability. J. occup. Med. *18:* 561–566 (1976).

MYERS, R.J.: Factors in interpreting mortality after retirement. J. Am. Stat. Ass. *49:* 499–509 (1954).

National Center for Health Statistics: Hypertension and hypertensive heart disease in adults, U.S., 1960–1962. PHS Publication No. 1000, Series 11, No. 13 (Vital and Health Statistics, Washington 1966a).

National Center for Health Statistics: Rheumatoid arthritis in adults, U.S., 1960–1962. PHS Publication No. 1000, Series 11, No. 17 (Vital and Health Statistics, Washington 1966b).

National Center for Health Statistics: Suicide in the U.S., 1950–1964. PHS Publication No. 1000, Series 20, No. 5 (Vital and Health Statistics, Washington 1967).

National Center for Health Statistics: Mortality from selected causes by marital status, U.S. PHS Publication No. 1000, Series 20, No. 8a and 8b (Vital and Health Statistics, Washington 1970).

NEUGARTEN, B.L. and DATAN, N.: The middle years; in ARIETI American handbook of psychiatry, vol. 1, pp. 592–608 (Basic Books, New York 1974).

OLIVE, L.E.; KELSEY, J.E.; VISSER, M.J., and DALY, R.T.: Moving as perceived by executives and their families. J. occup. Med. *18:* 546–550 (1976).

ORTH-GOMER, K.: Ischemic heart disease as result of psychosocial processes. Soc. Sci. Med. *8:* 39–45 (1974).

ORZACK, L.H.: Work as a 'central life interest' of professionals. Soc. Probl. *7:* 125–132 (1959).

OSTFELD, A.M. and SHEKELLE, R.B.: Psychological variables and blood pressure; in STAMLER, STAMLER and PULLMAN The epidemiology of hypertension, pp. 321–331 (Grune & Stratton, New York 1967).

PARKER, S. and KLEINER, R.J.: Mental illness in the urban Negro community (The Free Press, New York 1966).

PARKES, C.M.: The psychosomatic effects of bereavement; in HILL Modern trends in psychosomatic medicine, vol. 2, pp. 71–80 (Appleton-Century-Crofts, New York 1970).

PARKES, C.M.: Determinants of outcome following bereavement. Omega *6.* 303–323 (1975).

PARSONS, T.: Definitions of health, and illness in the light of American values and social structure; in JACO Patients, physicians, and illness, pp. 165–187 (The Free Press, Glencoe 1958).

PAYKEL, E.S.: Life stress and psychiatric disorders; in DOHRENWEND and DOHRENWEND Stressful life events: their nature and effects, pp. 135–149 (Wiley, New York 1974).

PEPITONE, A.: Self, social environment, and stress; in APPLEY and TRUMBULL Psychological stress, pp. 182–199 (Appleton-Century-Crofts, New York 1967).

PFLANZ, M.: Epidemiological and socio-cultural factors in the etiology of duodenal ulcer; in WEINER Duodenal ulcer Adv. psychosom. Med., vol. 6, pp. 121–151 (Karger, Basel 1971).

PINNEAU, S.R.: Effects of social support on occupational stresses and strains. Presented at a symposium on Job Demands and Worker Health. 84th Annual Convention of the American Psychological Association, Washington 1976.

PRIOR, I.A.M.; STANHOPE, J.M.; EVANS, J.G., and SALMOND, C.E.: The Tokelau Island migrant study. Int. J. Epidem. *3:* 225–232 (1974).

QUINN, R.P.; SEASHORE, S.; KAHN, R.; MANGIONE, T.; CAMPBELL, D.; STAINES, G., and MCCULLOUGH, M.: Survey of working conditions. Document No, 2916–0001 (US Government Printing Office, Washington 1971).

QUINN, R.P. and SHEPARD, L.H.: The 1972–73 quality of employment survey (The Institute for Social Research, The University of Michigan, Ann Arbor 1974).

RABKIN, J.G. and STRUENING, E.L.: Life events, stress, and illness. Science *194:* 1013–1020 (1976).

RAHE, R.H.: The pathway between subject's recent life changes and their near future illness reports. Representative results and methodological issues; in DOHRENWEND and DOHRENWEND Stressful life events: their nature and effects, pp. 73–86 (Wiley, New York 1974).

REEDER, L.G.; SCHRAMA, P.G.M., and DIRKEN, J.M.: Stress and cardiovascular health. An international cooperative study. Soc. Sci. Med. *7:* 573–584 (1973).

REICHSMAN, F.: Hunger and satiety in health and disease (Karger, Basel 1972).

REIM, B.; GLASS, D.C., and SINGER, J.E.: Behavioral consequences of exposure to uncontrollable and unpredictable noise. J. appl. soc. Psychol. *1:* 44–56 (1971).

REYNOLDS, R.C.: Community and occupational influences in stress at Cape Kennedy. Relationships to heart disease; in ELIOT Stress and the heart, pp. 33–49 (Futura, Mount Kisco 1974).

RICHARDSON, D.W.; HONOUR, A.J.; STOTT, F.H., and PICKERING, G.W.: Diurnal variations in blood pressure. Clin. Res. *12:* 57 (1964).

RILEY, M.W. and FONER, A.: Aging and society. An inventory of research findings, vol. 1 (Russell Sage Foundation, New York 1968).

ROBINSON, J.P.; ATHANASIOU, R., and HEAD, K.B.: Measures of occupational attitudes and occupational characteristics (Institute for Social Research, The University of Michigan, Ann Arbor 1969).

ROBINSON, J.P. and CONVERSE, P.E.: Social change reflected in the use of time; in CAMPBELL and CONVERSE The human meaning of social change, pp. 17–86 (Russell Sage Foundation, New York 1972).

ROMAN, J.A.: Cardiorespiratory functioning in flight. Aerospace Med. *34:* 322–337 (1963).

ROSENMAN, R.H.; BRAND, R.J.; JENKINS, C.D.; FRIEDMAN, M.; STRAUS, R., and WURM, M.: Coronary heart disease in the Western Collaborative Study. Final follow-up experience of 8½ years J. Am. med. Ass. *233:* 872–877 (1975).

RUBIN, R.T.: Biochemical and endocrine response to severe psychological stress; in GUNDERSON and RAHE Life stress and illness, pp. 227–241 (Thomas, Springfield 1974).

RUFF, G.E. and KORCHIN, S.J.: Adaptive stress behavior; in APPLEY and TRUMBULL Psychological stress, pp. 297–306 (Appleton-Century-Crofts, New York 1967).

RUSSEK, H.I.: Emotional stress and coronary heart disease in American physicians, dentists, and lawyers. Am. J. med. Sci. *243:* 716–725 (1962).

RYSER, C. and SHELDON, A.: Retirement and health. J. Am. Geriat. Soc. *17:* 180–190 (1969).

SACKETT, D.L. and HAYNES, R.B.: Compliance with therapeutic regimen (John Hopkins University Press, Baltimore 1976).

SALES, S.M.: Organizational role as a risk factor in coronary disease. Adm. Sci. q. *14:* 325–336 (1969).

SALES, S.M. and HOUSE, J.: Job dissatisfaction as a possible risk factor in coronary heart disease. J. chron. Dis. *23:* 861–873 (1971).

SAYLES, L. and STRAUSS, G.: Human behavior in organizations (Prentice-Hall, Euglewood Cliffs 1966).

SCHÄR, M.; REEDER, L.G., and DIRKEN, J.M.: Stress and cardiovascular health. An international cooperative study. II. The male population of a factory in Zurich. Soc. Sci. Med. *7:* 585–603 (1973).

SCOTCH, N.A.: Sociocultural factors in the epidemiology of Zulu hypertension. Am. J. publ. Hlth *53:* 1205–1213 (1963).

SCOTT, R. and HOWARD, A.: Models of stress; in LEVINE and SCOTCH Social stress, pp. 259–278 (Aldine, Chicago 1970).

SELLS, S.B.: On the nature of stress; in MCGRATH Social and psychological factors in stress, pp. 134–139 (Holt-Rinehart-Winston, New York 1970).

SHANAS, E.; TOWNSEND, P.; WEDDERBURN, O.; FRIBES, M.; MIETHOJ, P., and STEHOUWER, J.: Old people in three industrial societies (Atherton Press, New York 1968).

SHEKELLE, R.B.: Status inconsistency, mobility, and CHD. A reply to Horan and Gray. J. Hlth soc. Behav. *17:* 83–87 (1976).

SHEKELLE, R.B.; OSTFELD, A.M., and PAUL, O.: Social status and incidence or coronary heart disease. J. chron. Dis. *22:* 381–394 (1969).

SHEKELLE, R.B.; SCHOENBERGER, J.A., and STAMLER, J.: Correlates of the JAS Type A behavior pattern score. J. chron. Dis. *29:* 381–394 (1976).

SHEPHERD, R.J.: The influence of race and environment on ischaemic heart disease. Can. med. Ass. J. *111:* 1336–1340 (1974).

SMITH, H.P.R.: Heart rate of pilots flying aircraft on scheduled airline routes. Aerospace Med. *38:* 1117–1119 (1967).

STAHL, S.M.: Illness among the aged. A study of the determinants of the perception of the levels of health in an indigent urban population; unpubl. Ph.D. diss. University of Illinois, Urbana (1970).

STAHL, S.M.; GRIM, C.E.; DONALD, C., and NEIKIRK, H.J.: A model for the social sciences and medicine. The case for hypertension. Soc. Sci. Med. *9:* 31–38 (1975).

STAMLER, J.; STAMLER, R.; RIEDLINGER, W.F.; ALGERA, G., and ROBERTS, R.H.: Hypertension screening of 1 million Americans. Community Hypertension Evaluation Clinic (CHEC) Program, 1973 through 1975. J. Am. med. Ass. *235:* 2299–2306 (1976).

STANHOPE, J.M. and PRIOR, I.A.M.: The Tokelau Migrant Study. Prevalence of various conditions before migration. Int. J. Epidem. *5:* 259–266 (1976).

STANLEY, J.: Improving experimental design and statistical analysis (Rand McNally, Chicago 1967).

STERLING, T.D. and WEINKMAN, J.J.: Smoking characteristics by type of employment. J. occup. Med. *18:* 743–754 (1976).

STERN, M.P.; FARQUHAR, J.W.; MACCOBY, N., and RUSSELL, S.H.: Results of a two-year health education campaign on dietary behavior. The Stanford Three Community Study. Circulation *54:* 826–833 (1976).

STRAUSS, G.: Workers: attitudes and adjustments. In the American Assembly, Columbia University: the worker and the job: coping with change, pp. 73–98 (Prentice-Hall, Englewood Cliffs 1974a).

STRAUSS, G.: Is there a blue-collar revolt against work? in O'TOOLE Work and the quality of life, pp. 40–69 (MIT Press, Cambridge 1974b).

STREIB, G.F. and SCHNEIDER, C.J.: Retirement in American society: impact and process (Cornell University Press, Ithaca 1971).

STROMBERG, G.J.; PEYMAN, H., and DOWD, J.E.: Migration and health: adaptation experiences of Iranian migrants to the city of Teheran. Soc. Sci. Med. *8:* 309–323 (1974).

STRUENING, E.L.; RABKIN, J.G., and PECK, H.B.: Migration and ethnic membership in relation to social problems; in BRODY Behavior in new environments, pp. 217–247 Sage Publications, Beverly Hills 1969).

SUCHMAN, E.A.: Social patterns of illness and medical care. J. Hlth hum. Behav. *6:* 2–16 (1965a).

SUCHMAN, E.A.: Stages of illness and medical care J. Hlth hum. Behav. *6:* 114–128 (1965b).

SUSSER, M.: Causes of peptic ulcer. A selective epidemiologic review. J. chron. Dis. *20:* 435–456 (1967).

SUSSER, M.: Causal thinking in the health sciences. Concepts and strategies of epidemiology (Oxford University Press, New York 1973).

SYME, S.L.: Behavioral factors associated with the etiology of physical disease. A social epidemiological approach. Am. J. publ. Hlth *64:* 1043–1045 (1974).

SYME, S.L. and BERKMAN, L.F.: Social class, susceptibility and sickness. Am. J. Epidem. *104:* 1–8 (1976).

TARNAPOLSKY, A. and MCLEAN, E.K.: Noise as a psychosomatic hazard; in HILL Modern trends in psychosomatic medicine, vol. 3, pp. 90–101 (Butterworths, London 1976).

TAUSKY, C. and PIEDMONT, E.B.: The meaning of work and unemployment: implications for mental health. Int. J. soc. Psychiat. *14:* 44–49 (1967/68).

THEORELL, T. and FLODERUS-MYRHED, B.: 'Workload' and risk of myocardial infarction. A prospective psychosocial analysis. Int. J. Epidem. *6:* 17–21 (1977).

THEORELL, T. and RAHE, R.: Behavior and life satisfactions characteristics of Swedish subjects with myocardial infarction. J. chron. Dis. *25:* 139–147 (1972).

THOMPSON, W.E.; STREIB, G.F., and KOSA, J.: The effect of retirement on personal adjustment. A panel analysis. J. Geront. *15:* 165–169 (1960).

TWADDLE, A.C.: The concepts of the sick role and illness behavior; in LIPOWSKI Psychosocial aspects of physical illness. Adv. psychosom. Med., vol. 8, pp. 162–179 (Karger, Basel 1972).

TYHURST, J.S.; SALK, L., and KENNEDY, M.: Mortality, morbidity, and retirement. Am. J. publ. Hlth *47:* 1434–1444 (1957).

ULMAN, R. and ABERNETHY, J.D.: Blood pressure and length of stay in Australia of Italian immigrants in the Australian National Blood Pressure Study. Int. J. Epidem. *24:* 213–215 (1975).

VAN HARRISON, R.: Person-environment fit and job stress; in COOPER and PAYNE Stress at work (Wiley, New York, in press).

VAN ZONNERVELD, R.J. On measuring physical health in the elderly; in LOWENTHAL and ZILLI Colloquium on health and aging of the population, pp. 128–133 (Karger, Basel 1969).

WAN, T.: Status stress and morbidity. A sociological investigation of selected categories of work-limiting chronic condition. J. chron. Dis. *24:* 453–468 (1971).

WARD, A.W.M.: Mortality of bereavement. Br. med. J. *i:* 700–702 (1976).

WARDWELL, W.I. and BAHNSON, C.B.: Behavioral variables and myocardial infarction in the southeastern Connecticut Heart Study. J. chron. Dis. *26:* 447–461 (1973).

WARDWELL, W.I.; HYMAN, M., and BAHNSON, C.B.: Socio-environmental antecedents to coronary heart disease in 87 white males. Soc. Sci. Med. *2:* 165–183 (1968).

WEISSMAN, M.M. and PAYKEL, E.S.: Moving and depression in women. Society *9:* 24–28 (1972).

WEITZ, J.: Psychological research needs on the problems of human stress; in MCGRATH Social and psychological factors in stress, pp. 124–133 (Holt-Rinehart-Winston, New York 1970).

WERSHOW, H.J. and REINHART, G.: Life change and hospitalization – a heretical view. J. psychosom. Res. *18:* 393–401 (1974).
WESSEN, A.F.: The role of migrant studies in epidemiological research. Israel J. med. Scis *7:* 1584–1591 (1971).
WESSMAN, A.E.: A psychological inquiry into satisfaction and happiness; unpubl. doct. diss. Princeton University, Princeton (1956).
WHITE, K.L. and HENDERSON, M.M.: Epidemiology as a fundamental science (Oxford University Press, New York 1976).
WILLIAMS, C.A.: The relationship of occupational change to blood pressure, serum cholesterol, specific overt behavior pattern and coronary heart disease; unpubl. doct. diss. University of North Carolina, Chapel Hill (1968).
WILSON, W. Correlates of avowed happiness. Psychol. Bull. *67:* 294–306 (1967).
ZOHMAN, B.L.: Emotional factors in coronary disease. Geriatrics *28:* 110–119 (1973).
ZOLA, I.K.: Studying the decision to see a doctor. Review, critique, corrective; in LIPOWSKI Psychosocial aspects of physical illness. Adv. psychosom. Med., vol. 8, pp. 216–236 (Karger, Basel 1972).
ZYZANSKI, S.J. and JENKINS, C.D.: Basic dimensions within the coronary-prone behavior pattern. J. chron. Dis. *22:* 781–795 (1970).

STANISLAV V. KASL, Ph.D., Department of Epidemiology and Public Health, Yale University School of Medicine, *New Haven, CT 06510* (USA)